Rheumatism and Arthritis

What you should know about the problems and treatment

Malcolm Jayson is Professor of Rheumatology in the University of
Manchester. He formerly worked in the University of Bristol and the
Royal National Hospital for Rheumatic Diseases, Bath.

Allan Dixon is Consultant Physician in the Royal National Hospital for
Rheumatic Diseases and St Martin's Hospital in Bath.

Malcolm I. V. Jayson
and Allan St J. Dixon

Rheumatism and Arthritis

What you should know about the problems and treatment

line drawings by Gary James

Pan Original
Pan Books London and Sydney

First published 1974 by Pan Books Ltd,
Cavaye Place, London SW10 9PG
2nd printing (revised) 1976
5th printing (revised and expanded) 1979
6th printing 1980
© Malcolm I. V. Jayson and Allan St J. Dixon 1974, 1976, 1979
ISBN 0 330 23929 5
Set, printed and bound in Great Britain by
Cox & Wyman Ltd, Reading

to Judi and Sheila

Contents

Introduction

Why write a whole book on rheumatism ? Who other than hypo-chondriacs and doctors would want to read about it ? The answer is simple: we all get rheumatism in some form or another during our lives.

This book is written neither for doctors, nor for hypochondriacs to indulge in self-diagnosis. It is intended to fulfil a very real need for information. Rheumatism is one of the many medical problems where knowledge and understanding on the part of the patient make a lot of difference. Doctors are busy people; their time has to be spent on giving a correct diagnosis and recommending or prescribing the most suitable treatment. They do not always have time to explain what is being done and why. Many of the simple forms of rheumatism, such as sprains, cramp or a stiff neck, do not even involve a consultation with the doctor. This book describes what is happening or has happened, and its aim is to give a better understanding of why some things help and other things hinder progress.

However, the reasons for writing a book seldom coincide with the reasons for reading it. Why read about rheumatism ? Because it is so widespread; because it is a fascinating subject; because some forms of rheumatism have been the subject of remarkable advances in medical knowledge in the last few decades – and chiefly because the remaining forms of rheumatism still present major social problems with significant implications for all of us.

The word 'arthritis' means, literally, inflammation in a joint. The word 'rheumatism' is more vague, since it covers over 100 different conditions which cause disease of the joints or pain in the back or limbs on movement; some of these conditions are very serious, even life-threatening. But, most are relatively mild and more of a nuisance than a threat.

Sooner or later we all suffer from some form of rheumatism. Some forms, such as the stiffening of the spine and neck that occurs progressively with age, are so common that they must be considered almost normal. Indeed, we would be quite surprised if an old man of ninety was as supple as a young man of nineteen. Much of this stiffening process is painless, but there are often episodes along the pathway of a person's lifetime which are acutely painful. These are the lumbagos and painful stiff necks of adult life.

If rheumatism of this sort is in fact normal – and it is difficult to think otherwise since similar changes happen to animals and even the enormous dinosaur in the Museum of Natural History in London shows a similar stiffening in its spine – does it have an evolutionary purpose? The answer is probably 'yes'. Most features of individual animals throughout the animal kingdom are present because at some time they helped to ensure the survival of either the individual, the herd, or the procreation of the species. Man has descended from arboreal and nomadic ancestors. It is easy to see that an inability to climb trees or an inability to keep up with a tribe on the move would quickly rule out older members, who might otherwise continue to dominate the tribal family groups beyond the age of their maximum capacity. Now such activities are obsolete, and it is interesting to speculate whether rheumatism in the elderly still has a function. Perhaps a ninety-year-old labourer or managing director could cause a few problems!

Other intriguing thoughts follow. If we accept rheumatism as normal, then research into the causes and prevention of the 'normal' forms of rheumatism is really research into life itself. Perhaps it is a battle which will never ultimately be won, but even so, there are good reasons for not abandoning the fight. After all, a few lucky people have normal, or nearly normal, joints and spines throughout old age. In others these structures seem to wear out prematurely or just very painfully.

What are the differences between these people? Are they chemical – something to do with the actual composition of the bones and joints themselves? Are they differences in the way the body was originally constructed? Are we all basically the same, but some of us wear out more quickly through hard work, bad posture or poor nutrition ? Even if research cannot hope to provide us with the perfect, lasting joints, we can hope that it will explain how we can get better and longer use of those joints which we actually have.

The joints themselves are fascinating objects for research, although it is only relatively recently that medicine has taken a scientific interest in them. Other systems in the body are more dramatic. Stop the heart or lungs and Man dies within minutes. Research into heart or lung disease is much more appealing since it offers an obvious way of saving life. Damage the joints and the sufferer is crippled but he does not die. Research into joint disease has seemed less important in the past. But today we are learning, through research, how to control inflammation in joints and to replace severely damaged joints by spare-part surgery, just as we can replace kidneys and arteries.

Some of these advances have been so successful that certain diseases are no longer even talked about because they have disappeared. Tuberculous rheumatism, for example, along with the rest of tuberculosis, is practically non-existent in affluent countries. The reason is simple. We have learnt that this disease is spread by infected milk and so it has been possible to eliminate the sources of infection in milk supplies and to test herds of cows for signs of the disease. Everyone has heard of TT milk but how many realize that this means Tuberculin Tested ? And sufferers from the disease can now be cured by new anti-tuberculous antibiotics.

The virtual disappearance of rheumatic fever is another victory. With its complication, rheumatic heart disease, it used to kill 80,000 people a year in Britain, only twenty-five years ago. Now if it occurs it is usually in one of the mild forms which do not cause any lasting damage. Yet the organism which causes rheumatic fever is still with us. Known as the haemolytic streptococcus it still infects our children, causing them to have sore throats. Mysteriously, this is no longer followed by rheumatic fever. Some of the credit must go to the antibiotics like penicillin, but much must be due to better public health measures. At the moment we don't know which – clean water, clean food, less overcrowding, better diets – any or all of these may be important. The disease in its old and dangerous form is still present in less affluent countries such as in South America and India.

Research has led the way to important medical advances for some rheumatic conditions, but there are still more victories to win. Of these the greatest battle is undoubtedly with rheumatoid arthritis. This is, for many, a crippling form of rheumatism. It is also one of the commonest well-defined medical problems for which research has yet to provide cause or cure.

Cancer and heart disease, it is true, are more prevalent, but neither of these is just one disease. There are some forms of cancer and heart disease which are now curable. During your own life-time you, the reader, will have witnessed the triumphs of medical research in many killing or crippling diseases. Diabetes, pernicious anaemia, tuberculosis, syphilis, infantile paralysis (poliomyelitis) and a host of other infections have either disappeared or are treatable. By contrast, rheumatoid arthritis stubbornly remains unsolved.

These medical facts of life are at last being appreciated on a national and an international level, and are beginning to change the direction of public health resources. Until now the main effort of the World Health Organization has been on the great killing diseases – infections, heart disease and cancer. But increasingly it is realized that these are of less economic importance than the great crippling diseases such as arthritis and stroke. Although arthritis does not kill, it may prevent people from working and does not stop them from requiring medical help and economic aid.

In many countries the organization of the services to help those crippled with rheumatic diseases is still in its infancy. Some, however, are able to offer more than others in what they can do for sufferers. Disability is, after all, relative. A man in the middle of Africa is severely disabled if he is short-sighted and has lost his glasses. In the middle of London there would be no problem – he could go into any optician and get some more. Similarly, people disabled by rheumatism can lead perfectly normal lives in countries where the means and aids are there to help them.

Apart from help given to those already affected, there is an enormous amount of research being carried out into such problems as rheumatoid arthritis. Rough calculations show that over £200 million is spent each year throughout the world on research which is directly or indirectly related to this problem. It does not seem possible that the disease can resist research for many more years. Then at last we shall see another great victory in the battle against rheumatism.

1979

1 Our shared inheritance

Backache is one of the curses of man and, like all curses, a legend has emerged in explanation. The legend relates that, when man the hunter first began to attack and kill the animals of the forest, these creatures arranged a meeting to discuss defensive tactics. Each animal decided to curse man with a disease. The pig who loved eating gave him indigestion; the sheep declared that he should live without hair; the horse that he should walk on two legs only; and the antelope, a graceful runner, that man should get rheumatism in his joints!

But legends aside, backache is both a very old problem and a very common one. Examination of skeletons of ancient Egyptian mummies has provided evidence of problems similar to those of today, and the commonness of backache today must surely be self-evident.

Actual figures show that more than fifty per cent of all adults suffer from attacks of back pain. Every year in Britain, 35 million working days are lost because of rheumatic diseases – and of these the commonest single complaint is backache. The days lost to industry due to rheumatism are several times the total number of lost days resulting from strikes and industrial disputes. So, strange as it may sound, back troubles play an important part in national economy.

The structure of the spine

The fact that many different problems develop in the back is not surprising when considered in relation to the structure of the spine. It has to bear the weight of the body and yet be capable of bending and straightening for many years – such a construction would be considered a superb engineering achievement! The up-

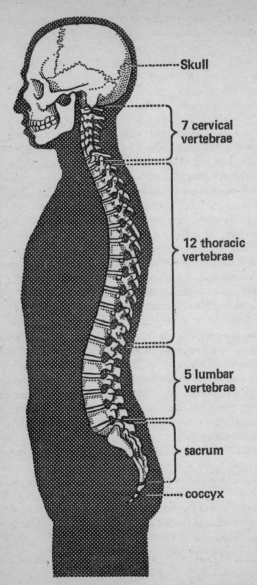

Skull

7 cervical vertebrae

12 thoracic vertebrae

5 lumbar vertebrae

sacrum

coccyx

The spinal column

right posture throws enormous strains on the spinal column and its associated ligaments and tendons.

The spine is a very complex structure and the principles of its construction must be clearly visualized in order to understand the various problems that produce back pain.

It consists of twenty-four blocks of bone called 'vertebrae' standing one on top of the other like a column of bricks. Seven of these are in the neck, twelve in the back of the chest, and five are in the low back or lumbar region. Beneath the lowest lumbar vertebra is a large triangular block of bone called the sacrum which is tilted downwards. Each vertebra possesses a cylindrical structure in front called the vertebral body and an arch behind, that protects the various nerves. The spinal cord leaves the brain at the base of the skull, runs down within these arches and divides into several smaller nerves which pass out through spaces between the individual bones.

Each vertebra is joined to the one above and below by an inter-vertebral disc and by joints. The disc is flat and biscuit-shaped, acting as a cushion, softening the impact of shocks and jolts through the spinal column. It has a soft, jelly like centre called the 'nucleus pulposus' and around the edge is a layer of thick, tough fibres called the 'annulus fibrosus'. These discs, despite having tremendous strength, also allow the column of vertebrae to bend and rotate. The vertebral arches are joined to those above and below by special joints.

On its own a column of vertebrae would be basically unstable, but the system is strengthened by the powerful muscles attached to its sides. Similarly the mast of a sailing boat is strengthened by the stays. However, a mast is not intended to bend. In the case of man, bending forwards induces the muscles to relax so that lifting weights from the floor can easily damage the spine. It is far better to bend at the knees and keep the spine upright – the muscles will then contract instead of relax and spinal damage is prevented.

The causes of backache

Backache is usually caused by problems arising directly within the spine. These are of four main types:

1 *Structural Change*. This can be a sudden mechanical problem

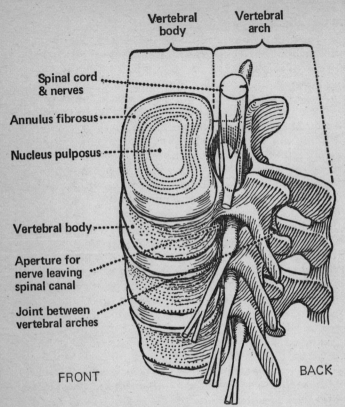

Typical lumbar vertebrae

such as in a prolapsed intervertebral disc (commonly known as a slipped disc) or it can result from 'wear and tear'. Also, occasionally, people are born with certain mechanical abnormalities of the spine.

2 *Inflammatory Disease*★. Inflammation can occur in the spine and may affect the joints in a way somewhat analogous to that of rheumatoid arthritis, or may be a result of an infection comparable to an abscess elsewhere.

★Categories 2, 3 and 4 are all dealt with in the next chapter

3 *Bone Disease**. The structure of the bone may be weakened and give rise to back pain.

4 *Tumours**. Growths of various sorts may occasionally occur in the spine and cause spinal damage and pain.

Most backaches, however, are due to mechanical changes in the spine (first category) and it is these that will be dealt with in this chapter.

Prolapsed intervertebral disc (slipped disc)

Previously, the intervertebral disc was shown to confer tremendous strength on the spinal column. This is true but, under certain circumstances, the central jelly like nucleus pulposus may burst through the annulus fibrosus. This causes the condition generally known as a slipped disc, but correctly it is called a prolapsed intervertebral disc. The distinction between these terms is significant. A slipped disc, the phrase with which we are so familiar, creates the wrong impression for it suggests that the whole disc slips and could perhaps slip back again into position. These implications obscure the actual situation – which is that the centre of the disc has burst through the outer ring.

Who is affected?

Prolapse of an intervertebral disc is most common in people between twenty and forty years old. The reason is that at this age the nucleus is most fluid. Later the central nucleus pulposus begins to dry up, becoming tough and fibrous and therefore less likely to extrude.

And yet another inequality reveals itself among the sexes – prolapse is more common in men than women! This difference, however, is not inherent in the backbones of male and female, but simply reflects the tendency in our society for men to undertake heavier manual work.

What happens?

The prolapse usually occurs at a weak point in the annulus fibrosus. This is commonly at the back of the disc towards one

* Categories 2, 3 and 4 are all dealt with in the next chapter

side or the other. When it happens, the disc contents are liable to press on one of the nerves that leave the spinal canal. The nerves may be merely irritated or suffer more severe damage, but the net result is pain in the area which that nerve supplies. Therefore although the pain originates in the low back or lumbar region – and is felt there first – if one of the nerves to a lower limb is pressed on, then the pain can also spread as far as the foot.

The nerves which join together to supply the lower limbs form the 'sciatic nerve' and hence this latter condition is known as SCIATICA.

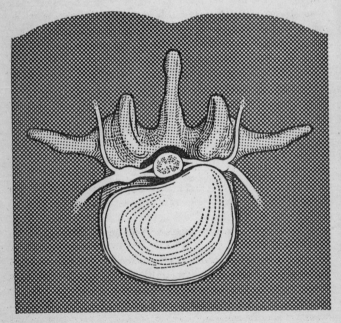

A prolapsed disc trapping a nerve

Although any of the discs in the spine may be affected, it is the lowest two discs that are most frequently involved, that is the discs between the two lowest lumbar vertebrae and the sacrum.

And why?

Prolapse usually occurs after strenuous exercise. The typical victim is the office worker who lives soft all week, sitting at a desk or in an armchair and travelling by car or train every day. Then the weekend comes and he attacks the garden or the house, or an exhilarating game of squash or golf is exchanged for previously non-active pastimes, such as reading the newspaper with his feet up. In other words, it is the unaccustomed exercise which initiates intervertebral disc prolapse.

The onset

The pain which is felt at the site of the disc protrusion is usually intense and sudden in onset. The sufferer feels as if he had been struck in the back but is unable to straighten up and look around. In Germany such attacks have earned the name 'Hexenschuss' which translated means 'witch's blow'. Sometimes the pain is so severe that the sufferer goes pale and may faint.

When one of the nerves is directly compressed, the pain spreads down the legs and sciatica develops – this usually appears within a few hours. The exact site of the pain depends upon which particular nerve is affected. Numbness or tingling may also develop along the area of the nerve and the muscles that the nerves supply may be weakened. Other ligaments in the spine can also be irritated and produce pain. This is felt as a persistent dull ache over the whole of the lower back and also in the legs.

Why are some people worse affected than others?

The reason for this is not only related to the amount of disc nucleus material squeezed out of its normal place and pressing on the nerves, but also related to variations in the amount of room available to accommodate the disc prolapse. Some people have large roomy spinal canals in which quite a large disc prolapse can occur without causing any serious damage. However, in others there is much less room and they get trouble more easily (see Chapter 2 page 60 for details of 'Spinal Stenosis'). Also, of course, there is always the natural variation in how much pain different people suffer from any particular problem. We all know people who say they never get a headache or indigestion. Probably we all get these things at some time, but some of us seem to have tough insides and don't feel much pain – or at least don't remember it. Others always seem to be complaining. Again, this doesn't mean that they are complaining of nothing. Their pains are real to them; they just feel them more easily than other people.

The symptoms

Patients with a prolapsed intervertebral disc not only suffer from great pain but are also unfortunate enough to resemble a rather stiff wooden puppet in their somewhat restricted movements! The difficulty in moving about and in bending the spine is created by the muscles in the back strongly contracting and producing a curvature of the spine. This is an automatic attempt by the body to reduce the pressure of the prolapse on the spinal nerves. Raising the leg by bending the hip and keeping the knee straight stretches the spinal nerves and aggravates the pain.

The doctor examines the patient to discover the areas of skin where there is loss of feeling and the muscles that have become too weak to show normal reflexes. All these changes reflect damage to the nerves and their consequent failure to function properly. The information collected will often enable the doctor to locate the exact disc which is at fault.

In many patients this is all that is needed to establish an accurate diagnosis. But sometimes it is necessary to rule out other problems and certainly in hospital a number of investigations will be done. Some of them, like the standard blood tests and x-rays of the back, can only give a limited amount of information. But there are new methods, including special x-rays in which fluids are injected into the spine, which are much more useful. They tend to be used when surgery is being considered. At present research is going on into even more sophisticated methods of investigation. One new technique is known as computerized axial tomography (or CAT for short!) in which x-rays are taken in directions which have never been possible before and allows detailed assessment of the size and shape of the spinal canal. There is another method using very high frequency sound waves, known as ultra-sonics, which provides some information about the size of the spinal canal and what is going wrong with it.

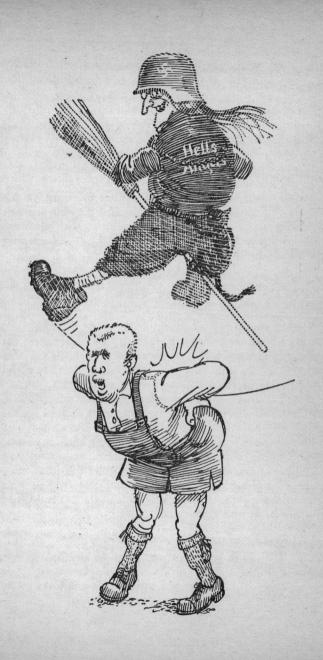

And the after-effects
Ninety per cent of all attacks clear up after a few weeks.
The pain and limitation of movement disappear whilst the
damaged nerves gradually recover. However, the outer fibres
of the intervertebral disc have been permanently damaged and
the central nucleus is very liable to prolapse again and cause
further trouble. For this reason, it is important to be careful not
to overstrain the spine again. Heavy lifting should be planned in
terms of the best and safest way – above all, weights should NOT
be lifted by bending the spine forwards.

Frequent relapses of a prolapsed disc are by no means uncommon. In time these will gradually diminish but, with permanent damage to the disc, the sufferer may be left with persistent
backache. Recurrent prolapse of an intervertebral disc frequently
progresses into LUMBAR SPONDYLOSIS.

Degenerative disease of the spine
(lumbar spondylosis)

When the young begin to age!
Any movable joint – human or mechanical – is liable to suffer from
'wear'. Most motor-car engines are discarded after only ten years
because they are worn out, but a human joint is less simple to
replace, and therefore has to last for many years.

Wear and tear of the lower spine is an example of a degenerative
disease which occurs in all of us. Its medical name is lumbar
spondylosis. Changes can be detected from the early age of
twenty-five years – and after that our spines can only deteriorate!
Contemplation of this fact incites the imagination to visualize a
world full of people with crooked spines and half-functioning
limbs. It is reassuring to know that fortunately many of these
changes do not produce significant problems and if they do, then
their effects are usually temporary.

The sufferers
Nevertheless some people, particularly those manual labourers
whose work involves heavy lifting, can become considerably – or
significantly – disabled. For example, coalminers and dockworkers

are more liable to develop lumbar spondylosis than office workers because of the heavy nature of their work. Furthermore, 'white collar' workers can continue their work despite back problems, but the same condition would incapacitate a manual labourer whose performance relies on the physical effort that he can produce.

What is lumbar spondylosis?

In this type of degenerative disease, wear and tear can affect both the intervertebral disc and the joints between the vertebral arches. The change is similar in both areas. The slippery cartilage

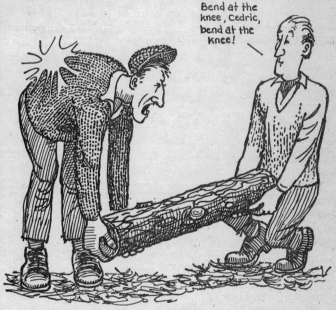

which lines the joint becomes damaged so that the surfaces of the bone become roughened and beaks of bone grow out from the side of the joint. These beaks develop as a sort of misguided effort by the joint at healing, but prevent the joint from moving through its full range. This helps to minimize the risk of further damage

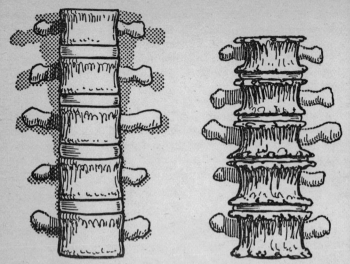

A normal mobile spine and a stiff spondylitic spine

but of course the loss of the normal range of movement – plus increased friction due to the roughened bone surface – means that the spine will become stiff.

Low backache
Lumbar spondylosis is the commonest cause of recurrent low back pain and backache. A persistent dull aching pain develops which is usually relieved by rest or by sitting upright with the back supported, and made worse by slouching in a chair or by doing heavy manual work. Occasional severe attacks of pain occur particularly after sudden exercise. The movements of the spine become stiff and restricted and a few unfortunate people with this type of backache often live a miserable existence due to chronic, persistent and recurrent backache.

Fibrositis or 'non-specific back pain'
Some people suffering from persistent backache are able to move quite freely, demonstrating a full range of movement of the spine.

The pain is often increased by poor posture when standing, or when sitting in a badly designed seat – such as in most modern cars. There may be tender nodules in the back and pressure on these aggravates the pain. X-ray of the spine is completely, or almost completely, normal.

Doctors use a wide selection of names for this condition such as fibrositis, postural backache, ligamentous strain, lumbosacral strain, sacroiliac strain, and so on. To be honest, these conditions are not understood at all and these names are largely derived from guesswork. There may, perhaps, be degenerative changes occurring in the spine which cannot be detected by x-rays or any other currently available types of investigation. Meanwhile, until research reveals the mysterious cause – or causes – of these conditions, it would seem preferable to be truthful and call them all 'non-specific back pain'.

In a recent study of over 300 patients with back pain sent to an Orthopaedic Department, the authors and their colleagues could only make a definite diagnosis for the cause of the pain in less than one in every two patients. Nevertheless, when these patients were seen at six months or more later, it was found that well over half of them had lost their pain – and it didn't seem to matter much what sort of treatment they had been given. So, here again, nature is coming to the rescue even when the doctors could not provide positive help.

Treatment and prevention of backache

There are many important points in the treatment of backache. The procedures used depend mainly on the severity of the pain, the extent of the disability and the cause of the problem. It is therefore helpful to consider all the aspects of treatment together.

Medicines to relieve pain
During the period of severe pain, the doctor will often prescribe strong drugs which may perhaps be given by injection. These are usually effective in relieving the symptoms but may have the additional effect of making the patient sleepy – this is perhaps not such a bad thing if he is confined to bed. However, some of these

drugs can be addictive and so should be stopped as soon as possible.

When the pain is less severe more commonplace drugs, such as aspirin, paracetamol, indomethacin, phenylbutazone and many others may be used. These medicines will be described in greater detail later, in the chapter on RHEUMATOID ARTHRITIS.

Confinement to bed

Complete bed rest is essential for sufferers in severe pain from a prolapsed intervertebral disc. The concept is, of course, totally unappealing, especially for those with active minds and bodies. But boredom is a small price to pay for relief of pain. People often struggle on for weeks or even months with severe backache before eventually accepting this advice. Complete bed rest in this context means lying flat all day, getting up only for meals, washing and going to the lavatory. Even these concessions are only allowed because they involve less effort than struggling with meal trays, blanket baths and bed pans!

Several weeks of rest in bed may be necessary before the symptoms disappear. But with strict adherence to these rules, many back problems improve within a few days. The rules can then be relaxed gradually and slowly the patient returns to normal living.

Choosing your bed – and lying on it

The type of bed is all important.

The criterion generally used for choosing a good bed is that it should be as soft as possible. But unfortunately this is a misleading fallacy – soft beds 'give' under the weight of the body with the result that the spine lies in a curved position during the night, aggravating backache. Many people suffer from backache in bed due to this very cause.

A firm bed which has a soft surface and yet provides full support is the best answer. This is where the quality of a bed comes in. A cheap bed has relatively few springs and sags easily whereas better beds have an increased number of springs which provide firmer support.

But for those of us whose financial situation imposes undesirable restrictions on such activities as buying expensive beds,

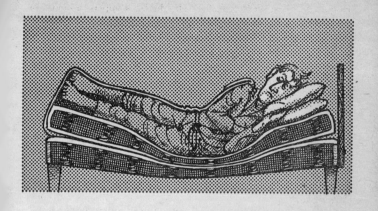

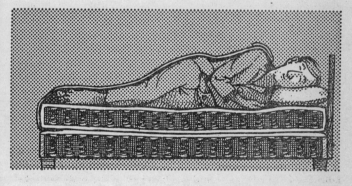

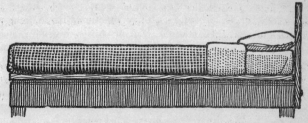

Beds – bad, good and improved with a bed board

there is a more economical answer. Placing a board beneath the mattress of the bed is a useful compromise and despite sounding rather austere, it is in fact quite comfortable. Three-quarter inch blockboard is best as it does not 'give' as easily as chip board and is still quite cheap. The board should be wide enough to support the full body and, of course, be as long as the sufferer. In double beds the board can be placed under only one half, but as this type of supported bed is not in the least bit uncomfortable, it is perhaps more conjugal for the board to be beneath both partners! Because of the size, two boards – one underneath each half of the mattress – should be used.

Sleeping as flat as possible with only one pillow will also help. Two or more pillows bend the neck, which in turn distorts the lower spine.

Many people who have been unable to obtain a good night's sleep for years have enjoyed complete relief by using these simple means – and once they have started using beds of this type they become habits for life. Even people without backache become aware that they sleep more soundly on a firm bed. An interesting fact to note here is that firm beds are generally used in the United States, and American visitors to Britain often complain of back trouble due to our soft beds.

Orthopaedic and other special beds

The term 'orthopaedic' refers to the kind of surgeon whose job it is to look after the problems of disease and injury to bones and joints. The word 'orthopaedic' itself means 'straight child' and so the orthopaedic surgeon originally had the job of correcting the deformities of crippled children and these were often the result of the long term effects of rickets. They sometimes had to break bent bones and reset them straight. Used in this connection the word 'orthopaedic' has some meaning, but the word is now used by manufacturers of beds, shoes and other devices to imply that there is some kind of medical approval attached to whatever they are trying to sell. It may be, as with beds, that there is nothing much special about them that isn't available from ordinary commercial ranges of beds of different hardnesses and costs.

When you buy a bed, choose it carefully to make sure it suits you. Firm beds are generally better than soft ones for people with back pain, but a 100 kg (220 lb) man obviously requires a different kind of springing in his bed when compared with say a 50 kg (110 lb) woman. If the bed suits you and it is what you want, buy it. Don't worry about the label 'orthopaedic' because that probably means you will have to pay a lot more for the same article.

There is another type of mattress which may be helpful to some back sufferers. It is filled with minute polythene beads and it is light and warm and can be changed in shape rather like a bean bag to fit exactly the hills and valleys of one's contour when lying in bed. Such bead mattresses are usually used on top of an ordinary mattress.

Spinal supports and corsets

Some people find it impossible to continue with a prolonged period of bed rest despite severe back pain. For them it is possible to immobilize the spine by use of a plaster-of-Paris jacket. This can only be applied by a skilled doctor or technician. The patient stands upright with the back in a good posture and the soft plaster is formed around the trunk. The plaster then dries hard and prevents movement of the spine. This is a less satisfactory method of resting the spine than confinement to bed, but nevertheless it is sometimes very useful.

In less serious illness, or if the patient still suffers from persistent mild low backache after the pain has become less severe, a lumbar corset can be of help. For this corset to be of any real value it must be tailored to fit the patient exactly. Those seen advertised in newspapers or magazines are of little use because they do not provide any rigid support and are not tailored to the individual person. A surgical corset of the required type contains steel strips running up the back. These are formed in the shape of the spine and restrict the forward movements that are so damaging to the back sufferer. A newer design of corset that seems promising employs a heat-mouldable plastic sheet instead of steel strips.

Lumbar supports of this type should be worn whenever there is a likelihood of strenuous activity. Some people find it best to wear their corset all day, but it is not often necessary to wear it during the night.

Attitudes towards corsets as being undignified and clumsy may unfortunately hinder some sufferers from using them, but a more practical problem is that many of these corsets are impermeable to air. This makes the patient feel hot, sweaty and uncomfortable. Lightweight air cell corsets can be obtained, but these tend to wear out sooner than the normal type.

Lumbar corsets should be prescribed by a doctor, the patient measured accurately and the corset supplied by a proper appliance fitter. Even after this, adjustments to the corsets may still be required to provide a satisfactory and comfortable fit.

The corset should be discarded as soon as possible, otherwise lack of movement may cause the spine to become stiff and the muscles to weaken and waste.

Sitting still and suffering

The rigours of an unpleasant sitting position are known to all of us. Many theatres, cinemas and particularly village halls seem to specialize in agonizingly uncomfortable seats which can convert a few hours of entertainment into an endurance test. This is particularly tortuous for the sufferer from back pain.

Certain basic points in the design of the chair must be borne in mind.

The purpose of a chair is of prime consideration. A reception chair in an office does not need to give the same extent of long-term comfort as that of the clerk. Although even this could be debated when remembering just how long it is often necessary to wait before being attended to!

A lot of research has been done into the most comfortable seats in various situations. It has become clear that there is no single ideal shape. A most important factor is to have sufficient room to change one's position from time to time. Of course in aeroplanes, where people are packed together to get as many as possible into the space available, the seating arrangements can make this difficult. But even here there is the facility for changing the angle of the back rest. If you are a back pain sufferer and have to travel by aeroplane particularly on long flights it is important to try not to sit too long in the same position. A small pillow in the low back is often a great help. Of course an ideal solution for those of us who can afford it may be to travel first-class in order to get the extra room.

In the office

The significant point here is that much more attention should be given to the design of office chairs, as clerical workers spend virtually all of their working lives sitting in them. The chair should be designed in relation to the accompanying working surface – it is better to think of the chair and desk as a unit rather than as two separate entities. There should be adequate leg clearance under the desk, and the lighting should be placed in a way that will not force the user to strain forwards out of a good sitting position and so nullify the design qualities of the chair.

The comfort of the chair is all important. Comfort, however, is subjectively assessed – the best solution would be individually designed chairs based on personal measurements and seating characteristics! But this is, of course, virtually impossible and chair manufacturers rely on standard information about the

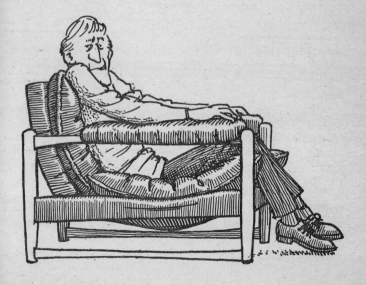

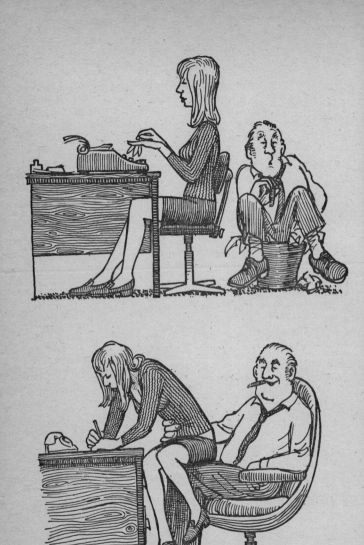

dimensions of the human frame. For office chairs, adjustments in height and degree of lumbar support should be provided.

At home

A common misconception surrounding ideas about a good comfortable easy chair at home is that low armchairs with soft cushioning and thick padding are the best, whereas in reality these chairs generate some of the greatest strains on the spine and are the least appropriate for sufferers from back pain. An upright chair with proper support for the low back is in fact very much more comfortable. A small pillow placed behind the low back will often improve the position in an otherwise unsuitable chair. The important thing is to restore the normal hollowing that should be present in the back.

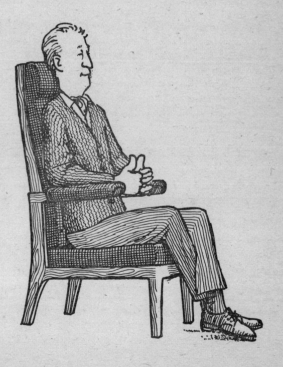

Padding and cushioning of a chair are important in preventing unnecessary pressure on the thighs and buttocks, but too much padding over a small area can restrict movement and lead to numbness of the skin. In order to avoid this it is essential to have a frequent change of posture.

And in the car

Equal attention must be paid to the design of car seats. These seats, particularly those found in certain small cars, are notorious for initiating problems in the spine. Commercial travellers are prone to backache because they spend long periods sitting still in a poor position. The ideal car seat should have an appropriate curve to fit the hollow of the back and be adjustable in both seat height and back rest angle to provide a range of comfortable positions.

New developments

An interesting point to note is that there are some significant developments in the design of chairs in Europe which will soon appear on the British market. Every time one sits down on a chair, the spine receives a blow. In this country this is softened by thick cushioning. In these new chairs, on the other hand, the cushioning is considerably thinner but the blow is counteracted by springing in the centre column or base of the chair.

The purpose of a chair is to permit one to sit and relax in comfort – and this should be the factor of prime importance when choosing one. Unfortunately, price, appearance and durability must also be considered, but this should never be allowed to persuade us to purchase a less comfortable chair.

Draughts and heat

A need to feel warm has long been associated with old people and rheumatism, and examples of this are obvious. Some people are particularly sensitive to the effects of cold, and state that their back troubles are intensified by sitting in a draught. They are unable to sleep at night without a hot water bottle, thick clothes or an electric heating pad to keep their backs warm. With this particular type of backache a woollen body belt or cummerbund may be beneficial.

Heat is a recognized form of therapy and warmth to the back is well known for providing a lot of relief. The simplest way of applying heat is by means of a hot water bottle. There is no virtue in this being too hot and certainly no need for it to be so hot as to cause any pain. A comfortable heat is all that is required.

Physiotherapists have at their disposal special electrical machines providing short wave diathermy or infra-red radiation which they use for treating some patients. These machines have the advantage of enabling heat to penetrate deep into the spine so that it is not expended on the surface of the skin.

Warmth and heat relieve pain at the time of application but in general it is unlikely that in the long term they would make any difference to the cause of the spinal disease.

Exercises for the spine

Recurrent attacks of back pain can cause the muscles of the spine to become weakened. Failure of these weak muscles properly to support the spine can in turn lead to the development of further damage. It is therefore important to preserve and restore the strength of these muscles. This is the reason for spinal exercises.

There is a wide variety of spinal problems and so the appropriate forms of treatment will differ. Some forms of exercise will suit one person's back but not another. The appropriate treatment is decided on medical advice but sometimes it is a matter of trial and error to find which is the most helpful. One form of treatment is to strengthen the muscles that straighten the back and arch the spine backwards. The back sufferer lies on the floor face downwards, hands by the sides, and attempts to lift the shoulders and chest off the floor using only the back muscles. Other forms of exercise include those aimed at restoring other movements of the spine and at strengthening the abdominal, or tummy, muscles.

An improved back, however, is no reason to relax – at this stage rather more vigorous exercises can be performed! It may be necessary later to restore the full range of forwards and sideways movements to the spine. But these exercises should only be performed under the skilled guidance of a trained physiotherapist.

It should be stated again (despite the fear of being tedious) that the right and wrong ways to bend must be remembered. When lifting a heavy weight, bend at the knees and keep the spine upright.

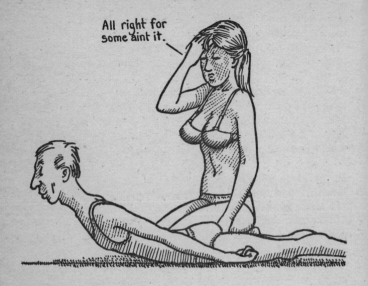

Massage and spinal traction

Massage is perhaps the most familiar and the most pleasant form of treatment of back pain. Repeated pressures are applied with the side or flat of the hand, softly at first and then with greater force. Massage is particularly applied to muscles in the back which are undergoing painful spasm, and usually provides temporary relief. Unfortunately, however, the benefit of massage does appear to be only temporary and when used alone it is of little real value. When massage has been applied to relieve spasm it should be followed by exercises which produce more permanent benefit.

Spinal traction, on the other hand, does not produce the same exotic image of treatment that massage elicits. Rather, stretching the spine sounds more like the medieval torture rack! Nevertheless, this stretching or 'spinal traction' can produce relief.

Originally, this method was applied in order to suck a prolapsed disc back into its appropriate position. Theoretically this sounds fine, but in practice it is known that it is not possible to pull the disc back in this way. Perhaps spinal traction frees a damaged nerve from adherent tissues or lessens the pressure on the nerve for, undoubtedly, relief can be obtained by these means.

Spinal traction is usually applied through a harness with the patient on a frame, but differs from the torture rack in that only small forces are applied, and these are carefully and precisely controlled. Sometimes the sufferer is put to bed with the foot of the bed raised about nine inches and traction is applied constantly using a small force. This has the advantage of combining traction with bed rest and relaxation.

Manipulation and osteopathy

Manipulation of the spine is a very controversial subject. The conditions so far described have all been due to mechanical damage and it would seem that these should be correctable by mechanical means. However, the spine is extremely complex and contains many delicate structures. Some patients improve considerably following manipulation by a skilled operator. Others, however, may be made worse. It is the basic difficulty in distinguishing the patients who would benefit from manipulation from those who may be made worse, which is at the centre of the whole controversy surrounding this form of treatment.

Manipulation, in this country, is applied by doctors, physiotherapists under medical direction, osteopaths and chiropractors. All four groups are highly skilled and have the ability to provide relief. However, careful examination of research data has shown that most backaches which are considered suitable for manipulation will get better by themselves within a few weeks. So that, although with manipulation, relief may be obtained sooner – perhaps immediately following the treatment – when assessed a few weeks later manipulated patients are not better off than those treated by simple means.

Osteopaths and chiropractors

The training of osteopaths and chiropractors is not along the orthodox lines of conventional medicine. The medical argument is that there is no virtue in being unorthodox – it simply means that many aspects of the subject have not been covered during training. Also that erroneous ideas about changes in the spine producing back pain can become accepted by the unorthodox without being challenged by critical observers, or by dissection at operation or post-mortem examination.

But to be fair, it should be added that osteopaths and chiropractors have displayed an extreme interest in patients with back pain who have often been neglected by conventional medicine. It is the failure of the medical profession to take a proper interest in this subject which has resulted in people seeking treatment from other sources despite the attendant risks and costs. With the current standards of medical care in this country, manipulation should only be undertaken by a skilled medical practitioner or by a physiotherapist under his direction.

Injections for backache

Various forms of injections are sometimes used for the relief of back pain. For example a direct injection of cortisone mixed with a local anaesthetic can often relieve the tender areas in the back.

In certain cases a specialist might give an injection directly into the spinal canal. This is known as an epidural injection and functions to displace mechanically the structures irritated by the disc prolapse. This may free a nerve which has been caught up with the edge of the disc and therefore provide relief from sciatica.

Surgery for a prolapsed intervertebral disc

In severe cases of disc prolapse, after there has been a failure to respond to the type of treatment previously described, surgery may be necessary. But this is, in fact, very rare. A thorough investigation is required in order to determine the exact site of damage to the disc. The operation exposes the prolapse which is then removed, together with the remains of the disc between the vertebral bodies, so as to prevent any recurrence.

This type of operation may lead to many weeks away from work and could prevent a manual labourer from ever returning to heavy physical employment.

Diet

Backache is not associated with any particular type of food, herbs or spice. You can, in fact, eat whatever you like – as long as you are not overweight! The logic of this is quite obvious really – being 15 kg (33 lb) overweight is the equivalent of a normal person permanently carrying a suitcase weighing 15 kg (33 lb). The excess weight places extra strains on the spine.

But, as most of us know from experience, dieting is easier said than done. Innumerable special diets from raw eggs to near-starvation are attempted for a few weeks and then abandoned in favour of less spartan living. It is more sensible and practical to make dieting part of a way of life. Once one accepts that certain foods are fattening and should always be avoided, then losing weight will be easier and more permanent. Bread, cakes, biscuits, sugar, sweets, chocolates, potatoes and all other carbohydrates should be eaten in restricted quantities. One of the authors has lost 10 kg (22 lb) in a few months on this sort of dietary regime.

Future research into back pain

Medical knowledge of back troubles is still incomplete. In many cases the exact cause of back pain is not fully understood and therefore research using many different techniques is needed to reveal the exact abnormality.

It is necessary to evaluate the type and amount of strain associated with normal muscle movements; mechanical calculations are being made to determine the size and scale of the forces to which the lumbar spine is subject during use; studies are being conducted to discover the mechanical strength of the body tissues; also, we have yet to find out whether there is any predisposing weakness in some of those people who suffer from spinal disease. The strength of the back depends upon its chemical structure and this in turn must be studied in relation to practical problems.

New methods of treatment for back pain are often suggested but these are difficult to test. The symptoms of back pain often come and go and so it is, in practice, often quite difficult to determine the true value of these treatments. Careful trials in clinical practice are needed to gain a better understanding.

2 Backache due to inflammation, bone disease and tumours

Most painful backs are due to the sorts of problem dealt with in the previous chapter. However, structural changes (such as prolapsed intervertebral disc, wear and tear disease of the spine, or strain of the various ligaments in the back) do not account for all back pains. In this chapter other causes of backache will be discussed. These are:

(a) Inflammatory disease such as ankylosing spondylitis
(b) Bone disease, infection and inborn abnormality
(c) Tumours

But even this list does not include all the possible causes of backache. In fact, not all back pain is due to problems arising within the spine; sometimes it is a result of disorders elsewhere, even though it is actually felt in the back. This is often termed 'referred pain' and is described later in the chapter.

Because backache can be attributed to such a variety of causes, it is important to be medically examined at the onset of problems. The character of the symptoms, the findings of the medical examination, and the study of x-rays and blood tests enable the doctor to distinguish between these different conditions.

Ankylosing spondylitis

Poker back

Ankylosing spondylitis is a very curious condition. The spine is first affected by backache which leads eventually to stiffening and an inability to bend. Even when the condition is painless – as it sometimes is – it can be exasperating for those afflicted by it, for the spine can become entirely rigid.

Ankylosing spondylitis has a very ancient and royal history. Sir

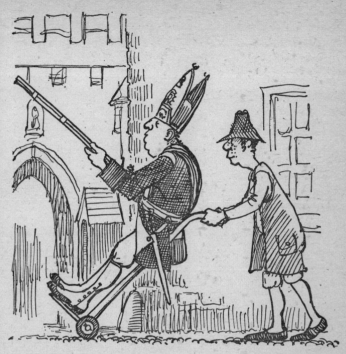

Grafton Elliot Smith in his excavations of the Egyptian mummies in the Valley of the Kings found several skeletons with spines typical of ankylosing spondylitis. In 1741 the Bishop of Cork described a man who was rigid from his head to his ankles. The only job he could do was to be a watchman in a sentry box, because he could only look in one direction and was unable to desert! Such a description could only relate to ankylosing spondylitis.

Victims of this disease may develop a characteristic – though unfortunate – posture; they may become intensely round-shouldered with such a bent back that looking straight ahead puts a constant strain on the neck. This is rare these days with proper treatment.

If the spine does become rigid but in a good upright posture the sufferer is not so badly handicapped, but even then he may have

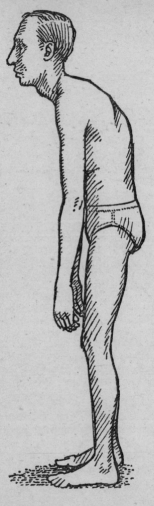

The posture in advanced ankylosing spondylitis

difficulty in looking to the right or left. This will interfere with such tasks as crossing the road or backing a car. Worse, however, is when the slouch develops to the stage where, when standing, the patient's head is pointing downwards to the ground.

From these descriptions it is easy to see how this disease has acquired the alternative name of 'poker back'. Modern treatment is aimed at keeping the spine mobile and the posture correct so that little severe disability should occur.

Who is affected?

Ankylosing spondylitis is not a rare condition. However, it is unusual in that, unlike some causes of backache, ankylosing spondylitis often affects a young age group. Because the first symptoms normally arise between the ages of fifteen and twenty-five years, persistent back troubles developing at this early age are quite commonly due to ankylosing spondylitis. This is particularly the experience of army doctors, who find that ankylosing spondylitis is a frequent cause of spinal rheumatism in soldiers.

Recent research indicates a ninety-per-cent or more relationship of ankylosing spondylitis with a certain blood group. In this case, it is not one of the familiar A, B or O groups associated with the red blood cells and which are important when considering blood transfusion, but one of the less well-known groups associated with the white blood cells. Knowledge of the white blood cell groups arose from their use in correct matching in transplanting organs such as kidneys. The white blood cell group involved in ankylosing spondylitis is known as HLA B27 and is inherited, so people born with this group have a much greater chance of developing the condition – six hundred times greater, in fact. However, at least four out of five people with HLA B27 never get ankylosing spondylitis. One out of five will get some form of it and of these most will be only mildly affected and perhaps never go to a doctor. Some physicians believe that an infection in the pelvis is the final trigger in a person who has inherited this susceptibility. Overall, only about three in every thousand men in the population, and even fewer women will get moderate or severe disease.

What happens?

Inflammation. The basic change occurring in this disease is called an 'Enthesopathy'. This means simply that there is inflammation at the entheses – the sites where the ligaments and tendons are joined to the bones. This inflammation then spreads to the joints, and particularly to those in the spine.

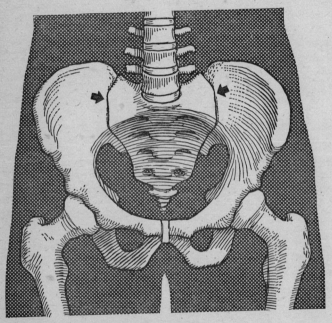

The sacroiliac joints where ankylosing spondylitis begins

The sacrum or tail bone is situated at the base of the spine and is joined to the pelvic girdle by the 'sacroiliac joints'. In ankylosing spondylitis inflammation starts in these joints and gradually spreads up the spine towards the neck. Sometimes other joints, particularly the hips, the knees and the bones in the feet, are affected.

A fundamental difference between ankylosing spondylitis and

rheumatoid arthritis is in the particular joints involved. In rheumatoid arthritis inflammation is concentrated on joints in the limbs and rarely affects the lower spine. In ankylosing spondylitis inflammation is in the spine and only later, if at all, affects the joints in the limbs.

Joint stiffness. You might think that inflammation of the joints is an unpleasant enough affliction. However, the real problem is the stiffness that develops as a result.

The site affected is where the capsule of the joint is attached to the bone. Bony outgrowths spread from the edges of the joint into the capsule. They eventually meet and so connect one joint to the next. The result finally is that the joint is no longer able to move. This is what actually happens in many of the spinal joints, and leads to the stiff 'poker back' characteristic of ankylosing spondylitis.

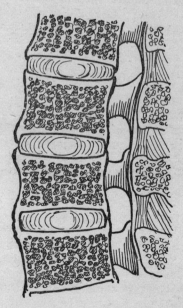

The sequence by which vertebrae become fixed together

Similar changes take place in the heel, for example. Pain and swelling at the site of the attachment of ligaments into the bone of the heel is eventually followed by bony spurs growing into the ligaments.

The symptoms

The onset. Ankylosing spondylitis usually starts with stiffness and pain in the low back. But a surprising aspect of this disease is that resting seems to intensify the stiffness and exercise provides relief.

It is very common to hear young men who suffer from this disease describing severe aching and stiffness in their backs during the early hours of the morning. They will often wake at 5.00 or 6.00 a.m., and as the disease progresses sometimes even earlier. Their tossing and turning in bed must be disturbing for any unfortunate wives, but it is even worse for the sufferers who are eventually forced to get out of bed in order to perform a few exercises. However, the almost immediate relief gained by standing up and touching the toes makes such an untimely activity worthwhile!

At this early stage, during the day the spine feels almost normal and a doctor's examination may reveal nothing unusual. Even an x-ray may not show any certain changes which could prove which disease the sufferer has.

For most people the disease burns itself out within five years or so, leaving them completely fit except, perhaps, for a little back stiffness. For a few, however, the disease progresses.

In more advanced stages of the disease, pain and stiffness persist into the day. Bending the spine is at all times both painful and limited – but this progression is not inevitable for all sufferers.

Sometimes other joints become involved. Inflammation of the hip or knee will lead to pain and swelling and may hinder normal movement. Inflammation around the heels has already been mentioned; this usually occurs beneath the heel, but sometimes the back of the heel is affected. These problems can make wearing shoes awkward and walking painful.

Severe ankylosing spondylitis. Inflammation gradually spreads up the spine and is reflected in the patient's inability to move easily. His movements become so restricted that he finds it difficult as well as painful to bend either forwards, sideways or to twist around. The difficulty – to use a cliché – becomes 'painfully obvious'! Instead of turning his head to look behind, the patient turns his whole body around, and if he needs to pick up an object from the floor then he is careful to lower himself by bending his knees rather than his spine.

Involvement of other joints has repeatedly been mentioned. The hips are most frequently affected, and if the spine is already stiff, this is a particularly serious complication. It is possible to move around with a stiff spine by using one's hips and knees, and alternatively, with stiff hips one is still capable of many activities using the movement of the spine and knees. But when both hips and spine are affected together, then the patient becomes severely disabled. Necessary activities, such as sitting in a chair or getting out of bed can, depending on the exact site of the stiffening, cause immense difficulties.

The joints which connect the ribs to the spine may also be affected. The same restriction of movement in the ribs means that the patient may have difficulty in taking a deep breath. The chest expansion on deep breathing is determined with a tape measure and tells how well the ribs move. In this disease the chest expansion may fall from the normal three inches to one inch or less. Fortunately, we breathe not only with our ribs but also with our diaphragms. In general, the diaphragm can compensate for the poor chest expansion.

Conditions associated with ankylosing spondylitis
Another peculiarity of ankylosing spondylitis is that it is sometimes accompanied by inflammation of other 'unassociated' organs in the body. Nobody knows why this should be – it is just a fact.
The eye. In front of the eye, the iris which surrounds the pupil, may become acutely inflamed. The eye feels painful and vision becomes blurred. Iritis, as it is called, occurs in about one-third of ankylosing spondylitic patients; sometimes mild, and at other times severe, it always has a tendency to recur. Proper treatment is essential in order to prevent damage to the eye.
The heart. Occasionally inflammation may also affect the heart.

This is focused around the aortic valve but fortunately it is quite a rare complication of ankylosing spondylitis.

The purpose of the aortic valve is to ensure that blood leaving the heart is pumped in the correct direction for distribution around the body. Inflammation in this area may cause the valve to develop a leak and fail to work at full efficiency, so that the functioning of the heart is impaired. In a few rare instances, it may be necessary for a heart surgeon to replace the aortic valve.

The bowels and intestines. Finally, revealing even more diversity in the associated effects, certain diseases of the bowels or intestines may also occasionally occur with ankylosing spondylitis. Ulcerative colitis and Crohn's Disease are two different forms of bowel inflammation producing diarrhoea and pain in the abdomen. The relation between these conditions – neither of which is fully understood – and ankylosing spondylitis has led to considerable speculation about the causes of these diseases.

Diagnosis – the importance of x-rays

The earliest changes are found in the sacroiliac joints where there are signs of damage, followed by bone spreading across the joint surfaces. Later these bony changes can be seen spreading up the various joints of the spine. Examination of the spine by x-rays is therefore essential for diagnosing early ankylosing spondylitis and reveals how far it has progressed in later disease.

Treatment

Keeping active

Physiotherapy, spinal exercises, posture. These must be emphasized again and again as being, without doubt, the most important form of treatment for ankylosing spondylitis. Treatment does not just come out of a bottle of tablets or from the end of a surgeon's knife.

It is only by performing exercises regularly under medical supervision and taking continual care with posture that the mobility of the spine can be maintained and deformity prevented. Infrequently performed physiotherapy exercises are not effective – they must be done every day for at least a quarter of an hour at a time. Twice a day is better.

The wisdom of this advice, however, does not always generate inspiration in the unenthusiastic! Boredom, lack of time, forgetfulness and laziness are all used as excuses to justify a lack of commitment, which sadly can lead to restricted spinal movement. Treatment of ankylosing spondylitis is, fundamentally, a constant fight to prevent the stiffening of the spine that characterizes the disease; frequent and regular exercise is the best way in which to fight this condition.

(1) The first group of exercises is designed to maintain the freedom in THE LUMBAR SPINE:

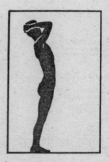

The patient stands with his feet apart, his spine arched backwards, with his hands above his head

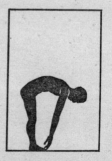

He then bends forwards and touches his toes

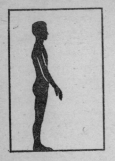

He straightens up, arches backwards and
REPEATS this TWELVE TIMES

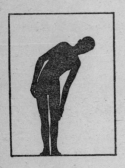

Standing with his feet together, he bends
his body to one side, sliding one arm down the
outside of his thigh towards the knee, and then
bends the other side of the body in the same
way. This again is performed TWELVE
TIMES

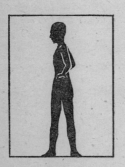

The final exercise for the lumbar spine it to
twist the body round so as to point one
shoulder backwards as far as possible. This is
performed first in one direction then the other
TWELVE TIMES

(2) A similar series of exercises should be done for THE NECK:

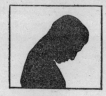

The neck is flexed forwards to bring the chin down onto the chest

It is then arched backwards as far as possible

The neck is flexed from side to side, bringing the ear down onto first one shoulder and then the other

It is then twisted in one direction and then the other, bringing the chin to each shoulder in turn

Finally, the head is moved in a circular movement involving all the joints in the neck

Each of these movements should be performed TWELVE TIMES.
(3) Further exercises are designed to maintain the movement of THE RIBS. These are quite simple: The patient takes a deep breath (using both his diaphragm and his ribs), holds it for a few seconds, and then breathes deeply out again.
(4) Exercises for all the other joints of the body have been designed making use of the full range of movement in each joint.

In particular, exercises for THE HIPS are stressed:

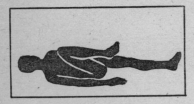

The patient lies flat on a bed and taking each hip in turn, bends first of all one knee up onto the chest and then straightens it

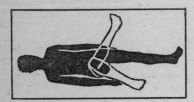

He bends the hip to a right angle and twists the leg outwards as far as possible, and then inwards

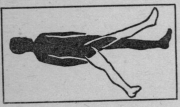

The leg is then placed straight out and the whole lower limb is moved horizontally outwards away from the other, and then inwards crossing it

All of these exercises are repeated TWELVE TIMES for each hip.
It is important to reiterate that the total period needed to perform all of these exercises is only about fifteen minutes and, if conscientiously repeated every day, they will prevent most of the trouble which arises in many ankylosing spondylitics. An energetic fifteen minutes each day is indeed a small price to pay for retaining movement in the spine.

Posture

The spondylitic should always be conscious of his posture when sitting, standing and walking. It is important to prevent a slouch developing. Instead the spine and the head should be erect.

The design of chairs is important, particularly for those who spend most of their working hours sitting at a desk. Spartan as it may sound, low armchairs should be avoided! An upright chair with some cushioning to support the lower lumbar spine is better.

Beds

A common problem already mentioned is the severe early morning aching and stiffness. A board under the mattress (of the same type as is used for people with prolapsed intervertebral discs) usually provides some relief.

Drugs

Drugs are of secondary importance in treating this disease. Their main value relates to the exercises – by providing relief from pain, exercises can then be performed more thoroughly.

Aspirin, indomethacin, phenylbutazone and other anti-inflammatory drugs are effective*, particularly for relieving early morning stiffness. A large dose of indomethacin taken at night as a suppository will also help relieve the stiffness normally felt first thing in the morning.

Cortisone and other steroids are rarely used for treating ankylosing spondylitis. Apart from not being very effective, they can have other, unwanted actions.

Radiotherapy or deep x-ray treatment used to be a popular form of treatment, but it has occasionally led to other complications and so now is rarely used.

Related diseases

Sacro-iliitis, or inflammation of the joints between the tail bone and the pelvis, is a characteristic feature of ankylosing spondylitis, yet is also associated with other diseases. The problem thus be-

* These are described in greater detail in the chapter on Rheumatoid Arthritis

comes one of definition. Because the changes in the spine are often identical with those in ankylosing spondylitis it is sometimes difficult to know whether the patient is suffering from ankylosing spondylitis plus the other disease, or whether they are just variations of a single condition.

Ulcerative Colitis and Crohn's Disease have already been mentioned as complicating ankylosing spondylitis. Similarly, it is well known that sacroiliac inflammation may complicate ulcerative colitis and Crohn's disease. Hence, it is the old question of which came first ? The difference between the two can be semantic.

Psoriasis is a common skin condition in which patches of thickened red scaly skin form, particularly over the elbows and knees. Again, spinal changes similar to ankylosing spondylitis develop.

Reiter's Syndrome is another, quite common form of inflammatory rheumatism. Similar spinal changes often occur in the development of this disease. Reiter's syndrome is sometimes a type of venereal disease.

Finally, *Still's Disease* (which basically is arthritis in children) is sometimes accompanied by sacroiliac inflammation. If Still's disease persists as the child grows up, the final picture is quite often that of ankylosing spondylitis.

These respective forms of arthritis are all dealt with in more detail elsewhere in this book.

Bacterial infections of the spine

Bacterial infections do not often get into bones, yet bacterial micro-organisms can occasionally invade and infect the spine in the same way as any other tissue in the body. Fortunately, such attacks in the spine are very rare but, when they occur, the spine can be severely damaged.

The infection causes inflammation which, when it affects the bone, is called 'osteomyelitis'. Also, if pus forms around the infected area, a spinal abscess will develop.

Severe pain, illness, a high temperature and shivering, are all manifestations of bacterial infections. Tuberculosis (which, mercifully, has now largely been eradicated) is caused by a special bacterium, the tubercle bacillus, usually affecting the lungs, but sometimes involving the bone, particularly the spine. This latter condition has earned the strange name of 'Pott's Disease' – for no other reason that than Sir Percival Pott (1713–88) was the first to describe it.

However, the near elimination of tuberculosis means that Pott's Disease is currently almost unknown. Bone tuberculosis used to be spread by milk from infected cows. Testing of dairy cattle and pasteurization of milk has been a victory of the public health service.

Brucellosis or undulant fever is also an infection transmitted in milk from cows. There has been an extensive campaign in recent times to eradicate brucellosis in the same way but it is still present in some dairy herds. Unfortunately brucellosis eradication does not seem quite as straightforward as the elimination of tuberculosis. Unpasteurized milk is liable to contain these bacteria and it seems that country living still has its disadvantages, for there is then a risk of catching this infection. Brucellosis is common in veterinary surgeons who have to deal with these animals.

The brucellosis bacterial micro-organism can become lodged in the spine or in the sacroiliac joints, producing severe pain and spinal damage.

All these different forms of infection are treated with modern antibiotics.

Abnormalities in the development of the spine

Another cause of back pain is related to the complexity of the spine. We expect errors to occur in the construction of a complicated artificial device, so we should not be surprised that abnormalities can occur in the development of such a complex natural structure as the spine.

The many vertebrae of the spine are joined by complicated joints and linked by a system of discs, ligaments and tendons; it is possible for any part of this structure to develop abnormally. For example, instead of having five lumbar vertebrae above the sacrum there may be only four, with the fifth one directly or perhaps only partly joined to the sacrum. Alternatively, there may be six lumbar vertebrae whilst the sacrum is correspondingly smaller.

These abnormalities are sometimes found when x-rays of the spine are performed on people with backache. However, the discovery of an abnormally developed spine is not at all as drastic as it sounds! In fact, it is usually of little consequence – this type of abnormality is found as frequently in people without back trouble as in people with back pains, only the former of course do not have their spines x-rayed. On the whole, unless they are very severe these abnormalities in development can be safely ignored.

Spinal stenosis

This is a gross abnormality of the shape of the spinal canal which has only recently received the attention it deserves. It is called 'spinal stenosis' because 'stenosis' means a narrowing or constriction. To understand its importance one must remember that the spinal cord and the nerves that come out from the spinal canal are suspended in a special liquid called the cerebro-spinal fluid. In a big roomy spinal canal, these structures are rather like apples floating in a barrel of water – very difficult to damage because they can float out of the way. But if the spinal canal is very narrow they will have no room to avoid a prolapsed disc if this occurs. Actually the space available within the spinal canal is greatest when it is slightly bent and least when the body is quite upright. This explains the experience of a recent patient. When she walked on the level her back pain became severe and her legs became weak but she could cycle up a hill without difficulty. When cycling, of course, the lower back is somewhat bent, whereas in walking she is upright and the back is slightly hollowed.

Spinal stenosis can be a developmental abnormality but, in some adults also it may be the result of bone disease.

Bone disease

Bone structure

Bone is a complicated material. Basically, it consists of an underlying mesh of tough fibres which are strong but lack any rigidity. The apparent rigidity of bone is derived from calcium in the form of a mineral called hydroxyapatite, crystals of which are packed

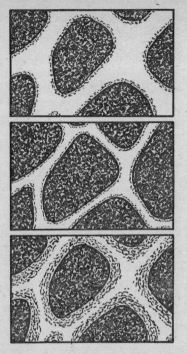

Normal bone framework

Osteoporosis – under-developed framework

Osteomalacia – normal framework but deficient calcium

like tiny bricks in this framework of soft fibres. The calcium is originally supplied in our food and reaches the bone from the blood. In order for the calcium to be properly absorbed into the body and manufactured into bones, there must be a sufficient amount of Vitamin D. This is the so-called 'sunshine vitamin', named, not because of any effect that it has but because it is formed directly in the body by the sunshine! Ready-made Vitamin D also occurs naturally in milk, butter, margarine, eggs and fish liver oils.

Osteoporosis and osteomalacia

The description of the structure of the bone correctly suggests that weaknesses of the bone are due to two main causes:

1 The first is that there may be a failure in the formation of the fibres forming the framework of the bone. A lack of fibres means that only a limited amount of calcium can be laid down on what is actually there. This condition is known as 'osteoporosis'.

2 On the other hand, there may be a normal amount of underlying framework but an insufficient deposit of calcium. The tissue therefore remains soft and is not converted into proper bone. This condition is called 'osteomalacia'.

Osteoporosis is quite common, especially in elderly people. More frequently seen in women than men, it is the reason for the stoop and loss of height which is a characteristic of ageing. Osteoporosis may also occur as a complication of other diseases and in particular may develop in patients who have been taking cortisone or other similar steroid drugs.

Osteomalacia tells a rather sadder story. It is due to deficiency of calcium and Vitamin D. In some of our cities the sun is hardly able to penetrate through the smoky atmosphere, so that the body is not able to produce the normal quantity of Vitamin D. If this is combined with an inadequate diet, osteomalacia is liable to develop. Again, it is the elderly that frequently suffer. This is because they have a tendency to live on the wrong sort of diet – tea, bread and jam – and often do not venture out of doors. At the other end of the scale, young babies in some communities are prone to this condition, although for them the disease involves other special features and is called 'rickets'.

Another reason for calcium deficiency relates to a rather complex chemical in food called phytic acid. This combines with calcium, making it unavailable for the bones. Phytic acid is contained in bread, but fortunately is destroyed by yeast during fermentation. However, it persists in unleavened bread and in oatmeal porridge and has recently been recognized as responsible for producing osteomalacia in racial groups accustomed to this sort of diet. A recent experiment of chapati-free diets for Asian immigrants has led to a noticeable improvement in the amount of calcium available for their bones.

For some people apparent lack of calcium and Vitamin D is caused by a failure to absorb these substances from the bowels. They often appear malnourished as other nutritious components of the diet are similarly not being absorbed.

If the bone is weak – or the load is heavy

Damage to the spine will occur if the heavy loads it has to support exceed the inherent strength of the bone, particularly if the bone structure is weak. Tiny fractures appear in the substance of the vertebral body causing sudden back pain. This can be incapacitating and is only relieved after a few weeks when the fracture heals. Recurring fractures of this kind can cause the height of the vertebra to decrease – if this happens to many vertebrae the sufferer appears to shrink.

Treatment

Only careful examination and blood tests will provide a distinction between osteoporosis and osteomalacia. Any obvious cause is then directly treated. Otherwise calcium and Vitamin D are given in carefully measured doses. This is successful in controlling osteomalacia but gives rather unreliable results for osteoporosis.

Acute attacks of pain in these conditions are due to small fractures in the vertebrae. This pain can be relieved by rest. For some it may be sufficient to avoid excessive exertion although in more severe cases, bed rest for a period, or a spinal support may be necessary. The difficulty, however, is that rest generates its own problems. Lack of exercise tends to result in the bones becoming even weaker, whilst using the spine tends to strengthen the bones. It seems to be one of those situations in which you can never really win! A vicious circle can develop: weakness of the bone leads to pain in the spine, which in turn leads to immobilization and further weakening of the bone. Any period of rest for osteoporosis or osteomalacia therefore must be for a strictly limited time.

Spinal tumours

Spinal tumours are rare, but a brief mention is necessary to complete the picture. They either develop in the spine or spread to the spine from other organs.

The tumours can be of two types. They may be benign, which means that they grow very slowly and can be removed without fear of recurrence; occasionally they may be part of a malignant cancer. Leukaemia and Hodgkin's Disease can sometimes affect the spine in this way.

Pain from the tumour is felt in the back. Also weakness or loss of sensation may be experienced in the lower part of the body if the spinal cord or nerve roots are damaged. Only careful examination and investigation can determine the existence of a tumour.

Paget's disease

Sir James Paget (1814–99) described a peculiar thickening of the bone which has since been named after him. This, in fact, is not a tumour, but is included here for want of a more pertinent place. The thickened bone has a rich blood supply and can occasionally be extremely painful. New drugs have been developed which are of value in controlling this condition.

Referred pain

At the start of this chapter, it was mentioned that not all pains in the back originate where they are felt. This is due to one of the peculiarities of the anatomy of the nerves in our body. When a particular nerve supplies several structures, irritation in one may lead to pain being experienced in another. An obvious example is squeezing the 'funny bone' of the elbow – this produces electric feelings spreading into the hand. The explanation for this is simply that the nerve running behind the elbow joint is being squashed.

Similarly, disorders in both the abdomen and the pelvis can produce pain in the back. Such conditions as peptic ulcer, inflammation of the pancreas and, within the pelvis, various women's diseases, may all produce back pain. Normally, however, there are other features or symptoms pointing to the fact that the primary disease does not lie within the spine. For example, with a gynaecological disease the pain is often related to menstrual periods.

To sum up

Most back pains are due to disc disease and wear and tear of the spine. However, there are many other possible causes, most of which have been mentioned in this chapter. Because of these different types of problems, each of which requires a different form of treatment, it is essential to identify the exact cause of the pain.

In conclusion, when backache appears for the first time medical advice should always be sought.

3 Neck pains

A pain in the neck!

It is not difficult to surmise how the phrase 'pain in the neck' became part of the English language. Both figurative and literal meanings of this phrase describe common intractable problems which frequently occur and which, although not serious, nevertheless produce considerable inconvenience. Neckache is common and troublesome and can affect almost anybody at any age. However, it is most likely to occur in the 30–50-year-old age-group. Although it is usually relatively mild, it can sometimes be both excruciating and disabling.

The structure of the neck

Before describing the different causes and types of neck pain, a brief outline of the structure of the spine in the neck is perhaps necessary to enable a clearer understanding of what can go wrong.

The vertebral column in the neck is similar to the rest of the spine, but differs in that it is designed for greater mobility and flexibility. The neck does not have to support the heavy loads which the lumbar spine must bear.

There are seven cervical (neck) vertebrae; these are all lightly built and the joints which connect each vertebra to the other allow for a relatively wide range of movements. These seven vertebrae stand on top of one another forming a column. As with the lumbar vertebrae, they have large cylindrical areas in front called the 'bodies' of the vertebrae and arches behind which protect the spinal cord. The uppermost cervical vertebra is joined to the base of the skull so that it is in intimate contact with the base of the brain. Between each vertebra there are small openings

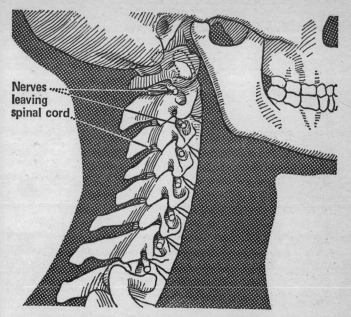

Nerves leaving spinal cord

The bones of the neck

through which the nerves pass out from the spinal cord to the limbs.

The two upper cervical vertebrae are more complex. The cylindrical body is missing from the top vertebra and is replaced by a peg pointing upwards from the body of the vertebra directly beneath it. This acts as a pivot allowing the head to rotate on the neck. The uppermost vertebra bears the weight of the skull and is therefore called the 'atlas' – an allusion to the giant who carried the world on his shoulders.

The vertebral bodies are joined to one another by intervertebral discs and the arches behind the spinal cord are connected by special joints. The structure of these discs is similar to those in the low back, consisting of a central gelatinous nucleus pulposus surrounded by a strong tough layer of fibres called the annulus fibrosus. The column of vertebrae is supported by innumerable ligaments and muscles. These impart tremendous strength to the neck whilst still allowing considerable mobility.

Cervical spondylosis

Wear and tear

The most frequent cause of pain and stiffness in the neck is wear and tear of the joints – so-called 'cervical spondylosis'. This is similar to lumbar spondylosis, which was explained in Chapter 1 and is one of the commonest causes of low back pain.

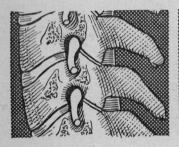 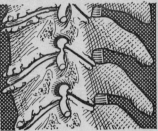

Normal vertebrae   Cervical spondylosis

Note how the nerve roots can be pinched by the bony changes in cervical spondylosis.

Wear and tear changes occur both in the intervertebral disc and also in the joints connecting the vertebral arches. The internal structure of the disc becomes deranged and slowly the substance of the disc is lost. The space between the bodies of adjacent vertebrae becomes considerably narrowed and the bone of the vertebra becomes thickened. Bony spurs called 'osteophytes' grow out around the edge of the intervertebral disc. Similar changes occur in the joints between the vertebral arches.

Stiffness

It is this damage to the joints and the emergence of the bony spurs that restrict the movement of the joints in the neck, with the obvious result that the neck feels stiff.

Pain

Pain may arise in the neck due to a variety of causes:

1 Pain may originate directly from the joints that have been damaged.

2 The various ligaments and tendons may be stretched because of the abnormal stiffness of the spine.

3 The osteophytes that are growing out from the joints may press on some of the nerve roots as they leave the spinal canal. This means that any movement of the neck can easily damage the nerve producing pain, not only in the neck but also in the area which the nerve supplies. As these particular nerves supply the shoulders and arms, it is those parts of the body which are most affected by this type of damage. If the precise site of the pain can be identified, then doctors can usually define which particular nerve root is involved. Nerve damage can produce sensations of numbness and tingling or the muscles can become weakened and lose their reflex responses.

4 In very severe cervical spondylosis the osteophytes project backwards behind the intervertebral disc and impinge directly on the spinal cord. This is definitely more than a 'pain in the neck' in both meanings of the phrase, for if the spinal cord is damaged there may be weakness and loss of feeling in the whole lower part of the body.

Do we all suffer?

It is a salutary thought that wear and tear changes in the neck begin at about the age of twenty-five years and from then on, as with the lumbar spine, the efficiency with which it functions gradually decreases. The inevitability of this process suggests that 'growing old gracefully' is a wise dictum, as by middle age virtually all spines show some evidence of wearing out!

So cervical spondylosis is very common, affecting almost all adults – it becomes more frequent with the progression of age.

Neck pains often start in the late 30s or early 40s. Usually the problem does not last more than a few days or weeks but in a few it may last much longer. Nevertheless, in virtually all sufferers the pains improve sooner or later. What seems to be happening is that around the age of 40 the discs in the neck are beginning to degenerate so putting strains on other structures. Later on, these other structures stiffen and will not move as much as they used to so that they are less liable to hurt. Of course in old age the neck is often very stiff indeed explaining why it is not common for very old people to complain of a painful neck.

Prolapsed cervical disc

A detailed explanation of a prolapsed lumbar intervertebral disc – popularly, but misleadingly, known as a slipped disc – was given in Chapter 1. It is also possible, but fortunately rare, for one of the intervertebral discs in the neck to burst or prolapse.

Accidents . . .

Accidents – especially car crashes – are the most frequent cause of this type of damage to the discs in the neck. The reason for this is that in most accidents, particularly in head-on collisions, the vehicle is brought to an extremely sudden halt; the driver's (or passenger's) body is held backwards, perhaps by a seat belt or the steering wheel, but the head is jerked forward by its own momentum. The rapid forwards movement is only prevented from continuing by the neck's attachment to the rest of the body, and after a sudden stretching the head is then rapidly whipped back, causing the neck to bend backwards. The head may oscillate backwards and forwards in this fashion for two or three times before eventually coming to rest.

Whiplash injuries of this type can produce severe damage in the neck (as well as other parts of the body) and an individual disc may burst in a similar way to that of a prolapsed lumbar disc. Headrests in cars are a safety measure designed to minimize the risk of this sort of accident.

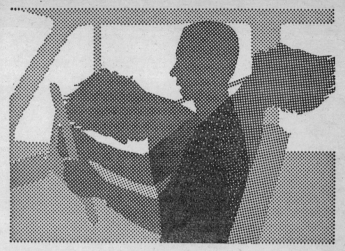

Whiplash neck injury

... Or bad luck?
Prolapse of a disc can, however, follow rather lesser injuries. It may be that there has been some previous abnormality of the disc which, by weakening it, has made it liable to burst.

The burst may occur to one side or the other and directly damage a nerve root, or more seriously may burst directly backwards and so damage the spinal cord.

... With unpleasant consequences
A prolapsed cervical disc generates severe pain and causes an extremely stiff neck. Sometimes, as a result of this, the neck is tilted to one side.

When the nerve root is damaged, pain, numbness or tingling may be felt in one of the arms, spreading to the back of the neck and perhaps into the scalp.

If the burst has damaged the spinal cord there can even be complete paralysis of all parts of the body beneath the prolapsed disc.

Cervical fibrositis

Pains in the neck have yet another similarity to pains in the back. This section refers to all those instances of people developing stiff or painful necks which arise for no obvious cause, and then disappear after a few days. This condition, termed cervical fibrositis, is entirely analogous to 'non-specific back pain'* and really just means pain in the neck for which there is no definable cause, nor anything seriously amiss.

Sometimes a stiff neck may develop after sitting in draughts, in people who appear to be particularly sensitive to the effects of cold and damp. It is also possible that there has been some strain to the ligaments or the tendons but neither clinical examination nor x-ray reveals any definable damage.

Neckache associated with other diseases

There are several other reasons why pain may develop in the neck, none of which, however, are very common.

Ankylosing Spondylitis, for example, can affect the neck. Occasionally the spinal symptoms spread all the way up the spine and reach the neck. If the disease is not properly treated, all movement of the neck may eventually be lost.

Rheumatoid Arthritis can also sometimes affect the neck.

Throat Infection or inflammation may occasionally spread backwards into the neck and produce neck pain.

Tumours of the spine are fortunately rare, but there are various diseases of the nerves that lead to neck pain.

Shingles (or *Herpes Zoster*, as it is correctly called in medical language) is a painful disease due to an infection from a virus which involves the nerves. When the nerves of the neck are affected, it is often difficult to trace the cause of the neck pain until finally a characteristic skin rash appears.

* For a description of 'non-specific back pain', see Chapter 1

Factors and conditions relating to neck pain

The most obvious causes of neck pain are damage within the cervical column due to injuries or any force that evokes a sudden twisting movement of the neck.

Poor posture when standing or too soft a bed for sleeping can also be responsible. Sitting at a desk which is so low that the subject is forced to have his head pointing downwards with his neck stretched will in a few hours lead to stiffness and aching. Properly designed office furniture should prevent much of this trouble.

Draught and damp have a peculiar penchant for producing pain and stiffness in the neck. This is a fact which experience will endorse yet, surprisingly, science cannot explain. A variety of possible causes have been suggested, such as stimulation of various nerves in the neck by the cold or the low barometric pressure, but this seems to be about as far as scientific knowledge has progressed.

The symptoms of wear and tear disease of the neck

Noisy joints

A distinctive symptom is the variety of clicking and grating noises that can be heard during movements of the neck. These noises are known medically as 'crepitus'. However, crepitus itself does not cause pain. It is produced by two roughened surfaces moving against each other. Crepitus from the upper neck joints is easiest to hear, as these joints are only a centimetre or so from the inner part of the ear.

Chronic aching

'Wear and tear' is often accompanied by aching, pain and stiffness in the neck. The pain is usually of a rather chronic, dull and persistent nature, although on occasions it may become intense for brief periods. It often spreads from the neck up into the back of the head or sideways into the shoulders and down the arm.

Stiffness

The movement of the neck may also be affected. The most marked change is stiffness when bending the neck forwards to lower the chin on to the chest. Also stiffness in turning from side to side can be particularly troublesome; this makes such activities as backing a car awkward for it is difficult to look obliquely backwards out of the window.

Aching arms and shoulders

Earlier in this chapter it was explained that some prolapsed discs may affect the nerve roots. This will cause pain to spread from the neck into the shoulder and down the arm. It is a paradox that in some cases there is no neck pain at all; only careful examination by a doctor will reveal the true cause.

Painful awakenings

Stiff necks are often made worse during the night. Long recumbency in one position (particularly if the neck is bent sharply because of the height of two or three pillows) can be responsible. A soft mattress increases the tendency to awake with a stiff neck because it leads to sagging of the spine under the weight of the body. The sufferer wakes up feeling dreadful with a stiff neck and has to wait for some time before the neck 'gets going' again.

Many of these night symptoms can be reduced by sleeping on a firm bed (as for low back pain) and using only one pillow. There are specially designed pillows with a thin strip down the centre so that they are in the form of a butterfly; these allow the neck to lie in line with the rest of the body.

Treatment

Most stiff necks – in fact, as many as ninety per cent – will get better without the need of any special medical treatment. All that is necessary is to keep the patient as comfortable as possible.

Heat and warmth

It was stated earlier that there is no scientific explanation for cold and damp having a tendency to increase neck pain. Similarly, it is not understood why warming the neck should provide relief – but it does! Tense, knotted up muscles seem to relax readily under gentle heat.

Heat can be provided through a variety of methods. Even a simple woollen scarf giving local warmth and heat to the neck will alleviate most stiff necks; a hot water bottle (not so hot that it burns) placed at the back of the neck will also help a lot; radiant heat from an electric fire can do the same thing, but again it is important to be very careful not to let the neck burn.

Physiotherapists have rather more sophisticated apparatus for producing heat. In particular, they use the short wave diathermy and infra-red radiation machines. In essence, however, the results (which after all is what it is all about) are very similar.

Massage
There is no need to explain how soothing and relaxing a gentle massage on the neck and shoulder muscles can be after a tense or busy day at work.

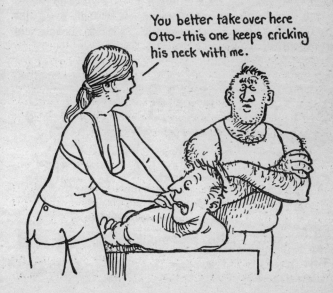

When a patient is in severe pain, the muscles become very tense and rigid which of course increases his discomfort; skilful massage can relax the muscles and certainly provides considerable relief at the time. But pleasant as this form of treatment might be, in the long run massage does not seem to make much difference to the progress of a painful neck.

Medicine

Because most stiff necks are usually brief and temporary, pain-relieving tablets such as aspirin or paracetamol are used to tide the sufferer over the difficult period. The dosage should not exceed more than two tablets taken three times a day. If this leads to indigestion or other side effects or if the pain is not adequately controlled, then a doctor must be consulted.

Neck collars

If the stiffness or pain persists, a tremendous amount of relief can be provided by resting the neck in some sort of special collar. This limits the extent to which the neck can bend or turn and so permits the damaged joints to rest. Usually the symptoms begin to fade after only a few days of wearing the collar and the problem becomes less severe.

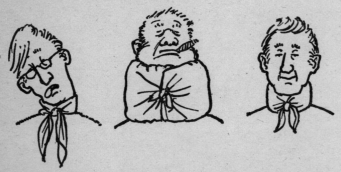

Not too little ... Not too much ... but just right

(Little Groping Parish Gazette) (New York Times) (Guardian)

The simplest form of collar can be made by anybody. It is a newspaper folded over, so as to make a strip about three inches wide and eighteen inches long and wrapped in a scarf. This should be tied around the neck tight enough to limit movement – but not so tight that it strangles the already stricken subject! The result is quite adequate for its purpose.

However, if that sounds too much like the Girl Guides' first aid methods, more sophisticated collars are provided by physiotherapists:

1 The softest collar consists of a thick layer of felt (of a similar type to carpet felt) enclosed within a special stocking. This hugs the neck closely and has the extra therapeutic value of providing local warmth to the neck as well as restricting movements.

2 More rigid collars are made of various plastic materials; recently new synthetic materials such as fibre glass, Plastizote, and low temperature heat-mouldable materials such as Orthoplast have been used as they show practical advantages over the traditional materials.

3 When it is necessary to wear the collar for a long period, special types are constructed with padding to prevent the collar rubbing against the skin, and with perforations to allow the air to circulate so that they do not become too hot and sweaty.

All these collars, although differing in their construction, share the same function – limiting the movement of the neck.

The Minerva collar, however, is entirely different both in construction and in function. It is used for only 0.01 per cent of cases and is especially designed for people either with a severe disease of the neck or who are recovering from an operation and require the neck to be fixed absolutely rigid. The whole skull and neck down to the shoulders are encased in a plaster cast.

Manipulation

Stretching of the neck is sometimes used as a form of treatment. The aim of stretching or traction is to relieve the pressure on the various internal structures of the neck that have been irritated. This is a delicate manoeuvre which requires a skilled technique and should only be applied by a qualified physician or physiotherapist.

Traction can be applied manually by grasping the head and pulling it very carefully in the required direction. Or it can be applied by means of a harness on the head and trunk. It is obvious that extreme care is necessary in order to avoid damaging the internal structures of the neck.

The problems of neck manipulation are exactly the same as with disorders of the low back. Manipulation is applied by doctors, physiotherapists, osteopaths and chiropractors. There is little doubt that skilled manipulation will often rapidly relieve the acutely painful and stiff neck. However, it does not always do so, and sometimes it makes the condition worse. Forceful and sudden movements of the neck can damage the spinal cord or nerve roots with the risk of producing pain, loss of feeling or muscular weakness in either the arms or the lower part of the body. For this reason some doctors have become rather wary and doubtful as to the true value of this technique. It is impossible to be dogmatic about who is liable to benefit and who to suffer from manipulation and so it is essential that the patient should know that there is a certain risk involved, however small.

Osteopaths and chiropractors have developed special skills for manipulation of the neck. Their fervent belief in the value of manipulation has led them in the past to claim that they could cure not only local problems in the spine but also other diseases such as high blood pressure or asthma. It is the extravagance of these claims that has led these practitioners to fall into disrepute. It is only at the present time that research is being undertaken aimed at evaluating the techniques of manipulation.

Exercises

After the pain has subsided, the patient may be left with a stiff neck. The answer to this? Exercises. These will help restore the full range of movement, promote the strength of the muscles, break down localized areas of stiffness and help the neck as a whole to regain its normal function.

Each case requires individual medical consideration but in general the exercises described in Chapter 2 for ankylosing

spondylitis should be performed, but with one important difference. In ankylosing spondylitis the patient is encouraged to
move the neck as far and as hard as he can in an intensive effort
to increase the range of movement. In cervical spondylosis the
patient should only move the neck until he is limited by pain and
not attempt to force movements too far.

Surgery

The need for surgery for these problems in the neck is extremely
rare. A burst disc or an osteophyte in cervical spondylosis may
impinge on the spinal cord or on a nerve. An operation may then
be needed to relieve the pressure and to prevent permanent
damage developing.

Research into the neck

Knowledge of the malfunctioning – and the functioning – of the
neck is an area in which the frontiers of science still need to be
pushed back! Or to state that in a less dramatic way, our understanding of the degenerative diseases of the neck is still relatively
poor.

We need to know what initiates wear and tear damage in some
necks but not in others, and the precise mechanisms by which
this damage progresses and gives rise to the common symptoms.

This leads us on to requiring a more detailed knowledge of the
mechanical changes occurring in the spine during all movements. A detailed analysis of x-ray examinations of the moving
neck should be recorded on cine-film or on television magnetic
tape so that they can be repeatedly viewed and examined. So far
there have only been crude measurements of the amounts of
twisting which occur at different levels. Also, the stresses in the
different parts of the neck generated during movement have yet
to be analysed.

Treatment of pain in the neck is not based on scientific
knowledge, but on methods that practical experience has suggested might be successful. There is a need to understand
precisely what it is that provides relief when the neck is manipulated or exercised. And we need to know exactly why local heat

will relieve pain, aching and stiffness. Comparative experiments with different forms of treatment must be applied in order to evaluate which types of treatment are most useful and which patients are most likely to benefit.

4 Rheumatoid arthritis

The word 'arthritis' simply means inflammation of the joints. Rheumatoid arthritis is only one of several different kinds of arthritis and when severe it affects not only the joints but also many other parts of the body.

We are all familiar with inflammation when it attacks the skin and causes such painful conditions as boils – the affected parts become red, swollen, hot and painful. When it clears up it may leave a scar. Similarly, inflammation can affect the lining of the joints so that they too become hot, swollen and painful. The joint then becomes difficult to move and does not bend as far as it should. Eventually the joint may be considerably damaged and internal scarring may stop it moving freely. The most common cause of inflammation of this type occurring in several joints in one person is rheumatoid arthritis.

Before describing the symptoms of rheumatoid arthritis and its possible causes, there are four relevant questions to be dealt with:

1 How widespread is it?
2 Whom does it most commonly affect?
3 At what age does it begin?
4 What is the cause of rheumatoid arthritis?

How widespread is it?

Rheumatoid arthritis is a common condition. It affects something like one in every fifty of the adult population. This means that there are about 1,000,000 people in this country with the disease, but fortunately most of these people are only mildly affected. Indeed some have such a mild attack that they do not feel ill enough even to see their doctors. They notice temporary pain, and swelling in their joints, perhaps in their fingers, but after a few weeks or months the symptoms disappear and there is no further trouble. For others, however, the condition does not settle down and it is they who seek medical help from their family doctors. A minority of this group who are more seriously affected go on to develop severe deformities and become crippled. These are the sufferers who are usually referred to hospital by their doctors.

Who gets it?

Unlike the conditions so far dealt with in this book, rheumatoid arthritis is much more common in women than in men. For every man affected there are two or three women with this disease. The reason for this difference is not at all clear but it probably has something to do with the female sex chromosomes.

At what age?

Rheumatoid arthritis usually begins between the ages of thirty and sixty but there is evidence that it can start at – literally – any age. It has been recorded that the disease involved an infant of only nine months, and at the other extreme of life's span, the condition can develop for the first time in elderly people, even in those over the age of ninety!

What is the cause?

The cause of rheumatoid arthritis is still unknown. Scientists have developed a number of theories and of these there are three which are generally the most acceptable:

1 The first theory suggests that the body inadvertently alters its defence mechanisms so as to attack its own joint linings – the synovium. This explanation comes from the observation that the joint linings show changes which are similar to those seen in any part of the body in which an 'antibody' reaction is involved, as in resisting a virus.

To enlarge on this latter point: we are already familiar with the term 'immunity'. A person is unlikely to suffer more than one attack of measles – because after the first attack the body has developed resistance against the measles virus. This resistance is due to the development of antibodies to this particular infection and to the appearance in the blood of cells which have learned how to attack the invader. Once these changes are present, fresh measle viruses entering the body are immediately killed. The body has developed immunity to measles.

Immunity, therefore, has a very important task in the body. But it can be harmful, or even destructive, in other circumstances. People suffering from a severe kidney disease may develop similar antibodies against a transplanted kidney. These, ironically, kill the new kidney in the same way as they would kill infecting organisms. This happens even though the new kidney is essential for the person's life.

In rheumatoid arthritis, for some unaccountable reason, the body's defence mechanisms may react against the joint lining in a similar way. The joint lining becomes inflamed and damages the joint.

In most people with rheumatoid arthritis, a special protein appears in the blood and can be detected by suitable tests. It has been called the rheumatoid arthritis factor. Indeed, this is the basis of one of the diagnostic tests for rheumatoid arthritis. What is interesting in connection with the theory of altered immunity is that the rheumatoid arthritis factor is an antibody. However, it is not an antibody to the linings of the joint but it is an antibody to yet other antibodies! The reason why it occurs has yet to be explained. It is already clear that this rheumatoid arthritis factor cannot be blamed as the sole cause of rheumatoid arthritis. Indeed it may occur in other conditions seemingly unrelated to this disease. However, if a great deal of this material is present in the blood, it may cause some of the complications of rheumatoid arthritis.

The theory of altered immunity as a cause of rheumatoid arthritis does not fit all the facts. It is clear that immune reactions occur and are responsible for some of the clinical features, but they are not the basic cause of the disease. On the other hand, immune reactions assume a more fundamental importance in a rare condition called disseminated lupus erythematosus and are dealt with in more detail in the next chapter.

2 A second theory is that rheumatoid arthritis is directly caused by some type of persistent infection. There are a number of known infections in animals in which the invading organisms enter joints to produce inflammation which is similar in some respects to rheumatoid arthritis. Intensive studies are currently being made to determine whether rheumatoid arthritis in man could be due to a persistent infection of this type.

3 The third theory combines the other two. An infection alters the joint so much that the body no longer recognizes it as its own tissues. So it develops antibodies against the altered joint.

What happens?

The first noticeable changes – as the previous discussion of its possible causes implies – are swelling and inflammation of the lining of the joint – the synovium. This becomes abnormally thick and swollen due to the persistent inflammation, and eventually it grows and spreads over the surfaces of the joint. Here it can, if it goes on long enough, damage the underlying cartilage – which is the natural load-bearing surface of the joint. Eventually it 'eats' its way through, causing irreversible damage to the normal smooth slippery joint surface. The ligaments which

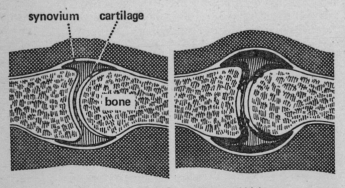

The synovium in normal and rheumatoid joints

provide stability to the joint are also weakened, so that not only is the efficiency of the joint greatly diminished but it also becomes unstable. Damage and pain can ensue because the joint is moved in directions or degrees for which it was not originally designed.

Movements can become so restricted due to the inflammation that the joint will only move through a part of its normal range; this is called a contracture. Or the alignment of the joint can be

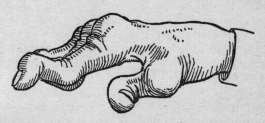

so disturbed that there is a partial or a full dislocation. In the case of the knees it may happen that the joint bends sideways to produce a knock-knee deformity.

Skin nodules
Inflammation can also occur in tissues under the skin, particularly in the forearms just below the elbow joint. This is the result of leaning forwards on the forearms when resting at a table. Small lumps called rheumatoid nodules develop which can grow and become tender.

Off-colour
Although rheumatoid arthritis principally affects the joints, it is important to remember that it is also a generalized disease affecting the total health of the person. This means that there may be changes elsewhere. The subject often feels off-colour, easily tired and very irritable. He or she is likely to have a slight temperature in the early stages and to lose weight.

Aches and pains
The first symptoms of arthritis are often just generalized aches

and pains, very similar in fact to those that develop during flu, but the difference is that they last much longer. Stiffness of the hands and the other joints is a common feature. This is particularly noticeable first thing in the morning and it may take several hours before the disabling effects of the stiffness subside. At this stage sufferers complain more of this than of pain.

Arthritis
Later with the further development of arthritis, the joints become swollen and painful; when pressed upon they feel tender and an attempt to use them generates pain. Because of this, the sufferer tries to avoid using the affected joints with the danger that movement becomes more and more restricted.

Which joints?
There are certain joints which are especially prone to be affected by rheumatoid arthritis. These are the finger joints (particularly those at the bases and in the middle of the fingers but not those towards the fingertips), the wrist joints, the knees and those at the bases of the toes. But, in fact, it is possible for any of the joints in the body that contain this particular lining tissue called synovial membrane – such as the ankles, elbows, shoulders and hips – to be involved, but these other joints are affected less frequently.

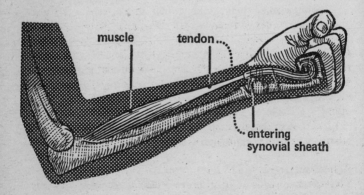

muscle   tendon...

entering
synovial sheath

And tendons?

The muscles supply the forces that 'operate' the joints by means of their leaders or tendons; these tendons are attached to the bones so that when muscles contract joints move. Because some of the tendons themselves run through sliding tunnels which are lined by a sheath of the same type of synovial membrane as the joints, they also can be affected.

This sheath may become so inflamed that scar tissue forms between the tendon and its tunnel. Consequently, the tendon movements become stiff, or the underlying tendon may be 'eaten' by this inflamed synovial membrane.

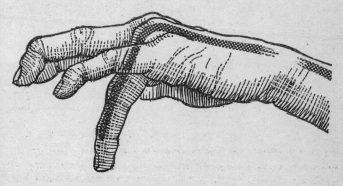

A dropped finger

Sometimes a tendon may actually become so weak that it will break and the particular movement can no longer be performed – the muscle is no longer connected with the bone that it is supposed to move. This is why some patients with rheumatoid arthritis develop a 'dropped finger'. The finger can grip but can no longer be straightened, due to a torn tendon at the back of the wrist.

Finally, a tendon may get displaced. When this happens, any attempt to move the joint increases the deformity.

What happens in severe arthritis?

Certain characteristic deformities develop in someone with

severe arthritis – you may perhaps have noticed them, for they usually involve the hands. The fingers may bend over sideways

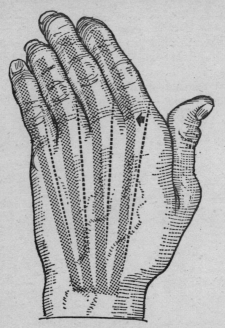

Displacement of the fingers sideways

and no longer remain in line with the forearm; or the finger joints themselves may become bent in various strange directions, so that it becomes difficult to use them. This is partly due to damage to the finger joints, but more often it reflects the displacement of tendons which pull the bones in the wrong directions.

Another problem is difficulty in bending or straightening the elbow. This may sound rather mundane but it is not. Imagine yourself finding it difficult to eat because you cannot put your hand to your mouth, or – even more frustrating – imagine not being able to scratch the back of your neck or do your hair.

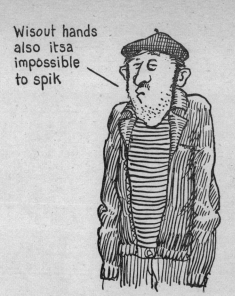

Wisout hands
also itsa
impossible
to spik

Another exasperating problem is when the joints at the base of the toes become severely involved – as they frequently do. These joints normally stand considerable pressure when walking or running. But when inflamed they become extremely tender; patients often describe the sensation as though they were continuously walking on pebbles or gravel. Later the toes get out of shape and the foot can no longer be fitted into a standard shoe shape. Specially made shoes may be needed to give space for the toes. In severe cases an operation to restore the foot shape can be very helpful.

Finally, there is an almost 'self-imposed' deformity: when the knees are badly affected by arthritis it is possible to obtain some relief when lying in bed by putting a pillow under the knees. This generates a terrible problem, for the knees may stiffen in the bent position. The result, of course, is that besides having developed an ugly and awkward posture, it is extremely difficult to walk. It is therefore imperative for patients with arthritis never to lie with pillows under their knees – the immediate relief

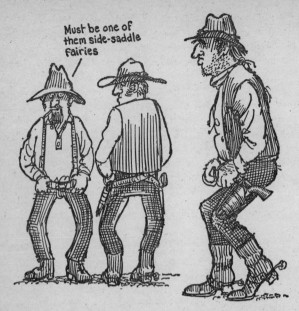

gained is just not worth the future problems. Special splints are made in hospital to rest the joints and prevent deformity of this sort.

It is far, far easier to prevent these deformities than to cure them once they have occurred.

Treatment

A massive research programme has been launched in the last few years in an attempt to determine the cause of rheumatoid arthritis. It is essential to discover if there is any infecting organism that might be responsible for the onset of the disease. Once the disease is initiated there is probably some sort of 'vicious circle' mechanism by which the inflammation becomes self-perpetuating, even when the original cause has long since disappeared. Some of the possible ways by which the mechanism might perpetuate itself are understood, but nothing is completely proved and many more scientific studies are needed. If this circle could be broken in some way, then perhaps the disease could be cured. Indeed the pace of medical research is such that we can reasonably hope to find the cure for rheumatoid arthritis one day.

But even if we cannot talk of a cure yet, there are several methods of treating this disease which are important as a means of providing relief from pain, preventing unnecessary deformities and enabling the sufferer to be as independent as possible. Because of the significance of these and because the disease is so frequent, these treatments will be discussed in some detail. They are divided into the following categories:

1 Rest
2 Occupational therapy, aids, appliances and adaptations to the home
3 Splints and plasters
4 Physiotherapy
5 Drugs
6 Surgery

1 The importance of rest

There is no doubt that periods of rest are of the greatest value to patients with rheumatoid arthritis. When the disease is really active and severe then complete bed rest is essential. People are often admitted to hospital purely for this reason alone. It is virtually impossible for some to obtain complete rest at home, as most young housewives with small children would agree.

Psychological factors are also important. Mental rest is equally as important as physical rest; being separated from the problems arising at home is just as valuable as the physical rest alone.

Confined to bed. At this particular stage, apart from getting up to go to the lavatory or to wash, the patient is 'confined to bed'. And this does not just mean lazily lying in bed all day. The position of the body in bed is important: the bed itself should be firm – with no sagging in the middle. The patient should lie flat and sleep with one or perhaps two pillows and, to repeat an

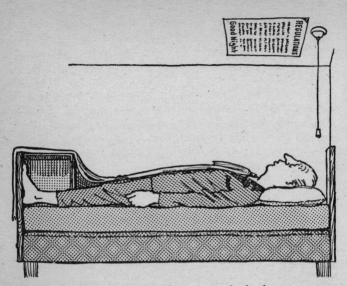

important earlier warning, pillows beneath the knees are em-
phatically forbidden. That may sound like a lot of regulations for
just lying in bed, but there are still more to come. If possible a
board should be provided at the foot of the bed for the feet to
press on, so as to keep the ankles at right angles to the body, and
prevent them from becoming bent pointing downwards. The
pressure of bedclothes on painful feet can create trouble and so a
cradle over the feet, under the bedclothes, is often used. If this is
not available at home, a large cardboard box, with two adjacent
sides removed is perhaps not as sophisticated, but it is just as
protective. Finally, when the patient sits up in bed, the back of
the neck should be properly supported by pillows.

Taking it easy. The period for complete bed rest of this type for
people with severe disease need only be two or three weeks. But
anybody suffering from rheumatoid arthritis should take a series
of rests throughout the day.

'Try to spend at least an hour extra in bed each night. Get up
late, put your feet up for an hour after lunch and go to bed early.
Avoid social commitments that would keep you out late at night.'

One of the best ways of starting the day for a rheumatoid arthritis sufferer is, like anyone else, with a cup of tea – but this should be brought to him or her at least an hour before she is due to rise and should be used to help swallow the first pain-relieving tablets of the day. By the time she gets up they will have begun to work. If she gets up with a warm bath, then much of the morning stiffness will ease up, leaving the joints in reasonable working order.

A word of caution is needed here. With early rheumatoid arthritis rest is helpful, often immediately and obviously so. With very late 'burnt out' rheumatoid arthritis rest can be overdone – the joints, though out of shape, need to be used and the muscles need to be kept in training just as in a person without arthritis. In the intermediate stages between early and 'burnt out' disease, it is often a matter of trial and error to see just how much rest and how much exercise are beneficial, and the guidance of the doctor or physiotherapist should be sought.

Remember also that the stiffness which comes on in the morning or after resting is not caused by the resting alone, and attempts should not be made to 'work it off' by vigorous exercise. Rather does it reflect the exercise of the previous day. So do not be afraid of extra rest periods. A short lie down after lunch can be the determining factor as to whether the sufferer can 'cope' with the afternoon or not.

Others need to understand the predicament of the sufferer and help when possible. This is particularly important for the patient who is both a housewife and mother; it should be appreciated by her family that she is no longer able to cope with much of the physical work involved in running the house. Other members of the family must help her with the shopping, the domestic chores and the younger children. Such help will lighten her burden considerably. If the family cannot assist or if there is no family, then the local authority will often supply home helps when there is a medical need of this sort.

2 The occupational therapist, aids, appliances and adaptations to the home

It is easy – but not practical – to believe that life can continue in the same way for sufferers as it did before the onset of the disease. That is not to say that rheumatoid arthritis should be seen as a crisis or a disaster, but should be recognized as a *real* situation which needs to be coped with through certain adaptations. The whole organization of the patient's daily life must be rethought. Living conditions can be designed to make life much easier for the sufferer. The occupational therapist from the hospital has received special training in this field, so it may help patients with arthritis to go and chat with her about their own particular problems. The occupational therapist may well want to visit the home with the patient to see actually what difficulties may be encountered, before she makes useful and helpful suggestions.

The kitchen, for example, is often poorly designed, forcing the poor housewife to walk many unnecessary miles during the day whilst carrying saucepans between the sink and the stove, and food between work surfaces and the larder. Simple rearrangement of the kitchen can help her considerably. For instance, the cooker should be next to a working surface or draining board and near to the sink, so that the housewife, if she has a heavy saucepan to empty, can slide it straight across from the cooker without having to lift it physically.

There is a wide variety of specially designed cooking utensils for patients with arthritic problems. For instance, if the patient has difficulty holding an ordinary knife because her fingers will not bend sufficiently to grip, then a knife with a specially fat handle may be the answer.

The lavatory can also be a problem. Patients with severe hip or knee diseases may have difficulty in getting on and off it. A simple grab rail and an adaptation to the bowl to give it a high seat may improve the situation. Another exasperating factor is that quite often the lavatory is virtually inaccessible, being up one or two flights of stairs which the patient finds impossible to climb. Today there are several models of completely hygienic and aesthetically acceptable chemical commodes, which can be wheeled to the patient and then stored away without any unpleasantness. A severely crippled patient may have great difficulty with personal hygiene after using the lavatory. For them a bidet with a spray followed by warm air for drying can be

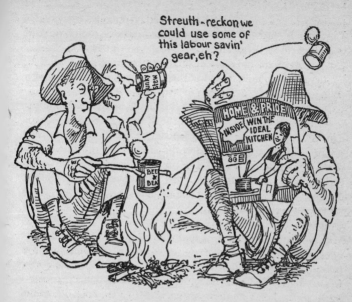

supplied. Likewise, a specially designed bath seat can be used if the patient has difficulty climbing in or out of the bath.

Even turning a door knob can be very difficult for a person with a weak hand. The most sensible suggestion is that these be replaced by lever-type door handles.

Combs with long handles, gadgets for turning difficult taps and devices for putting on and taking off stockings are all readily available. There is a wide range of aids and appliances for disabled people. If a disabled person has a problem, someone has almost certainly invented an answer to it.

People with deformed feet have enormous difficulty in getting comfortable footwear. Suitable shoes cannot be found in ordinary shoe shops and it is becoming increasingly difficult and expensive to have shoes made privately. Not having a shoe to fit the foot, in this country means essentially that it is impossible to go out of doors – slippers are no protection in this climate! There is now, however, a technique for taking plaster-of-Paris impressions of the feet and sending these impressions to a shoe factory which makes the shoes accordingly. The National Health Service will provide individually made shoes for those who require them for medical reasons.

A patient who has difficulty in getting around may also be helped by the simple method of using a stick or, in more severe disease, by the use of crutches or a walking-frame.

For many people these special aids, appliances and adaptations to the home do, in fact, represent the distinguishing line between dependence on others and independent living. As such, their importance must not be underestimated. They are just as important to arthritis as glasses are to the short sighted. All concerned with rheumatoid arthritis understand the problems involved and willingly give advice on all these points.

3 Splints and plasters

Just comfortably supporting an inflamed joint may provide a lot of relief from pain. In the early stages of rheumatoid arthritis in those few patients in whom the process is very severe, the doctor will often prescribe that the joint should be rested in a plaster-of-Paris splint. This applies particularly to the wrist, knee and ankle joints.

If the knee is badly damaged, problems may arise when the patient starts to walk again. A much stronger splint, made perhaps out of plastic, is then used to support the knee, enabling the patient to walk without the joint coming under strain until the muscles have recovered enough to hold the joint normally.

4 Physiotherapy

The purpose of physiotherapy is to maintain and improve the range of the movements of the joints and to increase the strength of the muscles which control them. Various exercises may be prescribed by the physician with these aims in mind.

Exercise. In the acute stage of the disease when all the joints are very inflamed and painful, attempting to perform powerful exercises is futile. They are just impossible for the patient to do. All that is necessary at this stage is to put the joint through a complete range of movements several times a day. It is very much easier if this is done by a friend or by a physiotherapist who can bear the weight of the leg, for example, so that the patient does not have to use his or her own muscles.

When the disease is less severe, then more active exercises with the patients doing the work themselves are necessary.

In the hand, for instance, a simple exercise of repeatedly clenching the fist and then straightening the fingers can be useful – for both regaining and retaining movements.

Similarly, the elbow should be bent and then straightened several times.

The shoulders can usefully be moved in a complete circle. The patient stands or sits upright and moves one shoulder at a time in all directions. If this is too painful a similar exercise can be done lying on a bed. Gravity then assists and it is easier to stretch the shoulder fully by reaching through the bars at the head of the bed.

Likewise, a wide range of movements in the hip and ankle joints should be practised.

Knee exercises are most important; the quadriceps muscle – that is the large muscle lying in front of the thigh – tends to waste away very rapidly when there is disease in the knee. It is

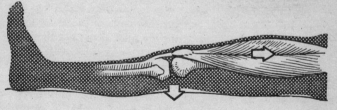

Quadriceps muscle

possible to prevent this to a considerable extent if the quadriceps muscle is exercised. The patient lies flat in bed and forcibly pushes the back of the knee downwards on to the bed, at the same time contracting the muscle and pulling up the knee cap. Another exercise is to lie flat in bed and raise the whole of the leg, keeping the knee as straight as possible. As the strength of the muscle improves, this exercise should be made harder by adding weights to the shin. The suggested way of doing this is to

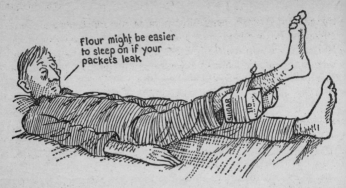

strap a couple of pound bags of sugar around the shin and then elevate the leg again with the knee straight! This may sound rather bizarre, but it does work.

These exercises should be performed for a period of about a quarter of an hour each time at least daily, but preferably twice a day. The problem is that exercises can be very tiring for arthritics, particularly if they involve lifting the weight of one's own limbs.

This latter situation is especially difficult for patients who have severe pain in the hip. Occasionally contraptions with slings and pulleys are rigged up to support the whole of the lower limb, enabling the patient to move the hip joint alone, but these are very difficult to organize at home.

Hydrotherapy. One way of coping with the weight of the limb is with the use of water. Physiotherapy exercises in water are therefore often prescribed. This is part of what is termed 'hydrotherapy'. Basically, these exercises are performed in a large shallow warm swimming pool. There is usually a slope on one side of the pool so that patients can walk down to the required depth. When in the pool the weight of the patient's body is considerably lighter (because it is under water) so the painful joint can be moved with much less effort. It is then very easy to do hip and other exercises. The physiotherapists that specialize in this type of therapy are called 'hydrotherapists'.

Of all the methods of getting stiff joints working again, hydrotherapy in a warm swimming pool is the most pleasant and effective. In the past the great spas and watering places of Europe built up their reputation partly on the results of treatment in swimming baths fed by natural hot springs. Spas and spa therapy are dealt with in more detail in Chapter 12.

Hydrotherapy, although beneficial in all except the early stages of rheumatoid arthritis, is also very tiring and should always be followed by a period of rest, the patient wrapped up in a large warm towel. And if hydrotherapy is prescribed for the morning, then nothing active should be planned for the afternoon or evening of that day.

Rheumatoid arthritis patients can often help themselves by performing these exercises in a public swimming pool. And if that sounds too conspicuous, there is no need to worry because even swimming itself is a very good exercise.

Heat. And if swimming seems an appealing type of therapy, 'heat' for the less active must surely sound even more attractive and comforting! Relief for a painful joint can often be obtained at home by sitting in front of a radiant electric fire or by placing a hot water bottle on the painful area – although it is, of course, essential to be careful not to burn the skin.

There are, however, more sophisticated methods of applying heat which appear to be somewhat more effective.

Wax baths are useful for the painful hand. A special grade of paraffin wax is used for this purpose and can be bought from the chemist. It is essential to use the right wax as other waxes melt at too high a temperature which would mean that if the hand was dipped into them, the skin would be severely burnt. When used at home, this wax should never be melted directly on an electric or gas fire for it can easily be overheated. It should be melted in a double saucepan so that it is gently steamed from beneath, and only heated to the temperature that is required just to melt it. The hand is dipped in and out of the wax about half a dozen times until it has a thick coating of warm wax around it. Then it is wrapped in cotton wool and bandages to preserve the heat. This will provide gentle heat in the inflamed area for about half an hour or more and it is possible to exercise the hand within the wax glove. At the end of this time the wax glove can be stripped off and returned for remelting.

In addition to wax baths, there is a variety of complex electrical apparatus which is used in hospitals for applying heat to inflamed joints. They have the advantage over domestic electric fires in that the heat penetrates deep into the tissues rather than being dissipated on the surface. The use of this apparatus, however, must be under the control of a trained physiotherapist.

5 Medical control of arthritis

The drugs used can be considered under six headings:

(a) Drugs that kill pain and suppress inflammation;
(b) Drugs that produce remissions of rheumatoid arthritis;
(c) Steroid and cortisone preparations;
(d) Drugs that suppress immunity;
(e) Drugs which help deal with complications of rheumatoid arthritis, such as anaemia;
(f) Radio-active injections;
(g) Research into drugs for rheumatoid arthritis.

(a) *Drugs relieving pain and inflammation*. We are all familiar with aspirin as a drug for relieving pain – and as such it is the most useful drug for treating rheumatoid arthritis. If taken in the full dosage it will actually suppress the inflammation; this has been proved by a very clever study in which the sizes of inflamed finger joints were measured using jewellers' rings. This means patients must consult their doctor, agree on an appropriate dosage and then stick to it.

But every medicament known to physicians can produce undesirable side effects. Aspirin is no exception, but it is on the whole a fairly safe drug. Many tons of aspirin are consumed every year in this country and yet the frequency of side effects remains very low.

One of the possible problems with aspirin is that it is liable to produce indigestion and stomach pains. If this develops, the doctor must be consulted for advice as to whether the drug be stopped. There are some specially prepared formulations and derivatives of aspirin available. Some of these have a protective coating on them which helps to prevent the aspirin from irritating the stomach lining.

Another disadvantage of aspirin is the number of tablets that have to be taken – twelve or more a day sometimes. There is now a liquid form of aspirin which is only taken two or three times a day for the same effect.

Alternative available drugs which similarly reduce pain and suppress inflammation are indomethacin (Indocid), phenylbutazone (Butazolidin), ibuprofen (Brufen), naproxen (Naprosyn) and many others. Indomethacin causes headaches in some people and can occasionally produce the same sort of indigestion problems as aspirin. Phenylbutazone may sometimes produce severe stomach ulcers and, rarely, disturbances in the blood which can be serious. Any patients taking these drugs should be regularly reviewed by their doctors.

Paracetamol (Panadol) appears to be a rather innocuous drug which has hardly ever produced any unwanted side effects, but it does not appear to be nearly as effective as the other agents.

Phenacetin must be mentioned in terms of a warning. This is a drug which is particularly effective in relieving pain, but unfortunately if it is taken for many years it can lead to severe kidney damage. It should be avoided completely by patients with arthritis, some of whom need to take tablets daily indefinitely. Phenacetin is not usually sold as an isolated drug but is often present as one of a mixture of compounds presented under various trade names. The commonest of these contain aspirin, phenacetin and codeine and are often called 'Codeine tablets'. Because of the problems that may arise, tablets containing phenacetin are no longer freely available in Britain, although they may be obtained elsewhere. Any arthritic purchasing tablets must ask the pharmacist or else read the small print on the container to make sure that no phenacetin is present.

(b) *Drugs that produce remissions of rheumatoid arthritis.* There are certain drugs which function not to relieve pain and inflammation in the same way as aspirin, but to encourage a remission – or a 'clearing up' – of the disease two or three months after the start of the treatment. They are the nearest thing which medicine has to a cure of the disease. Unfortunately, they do not work in all cases, nor can the benefit be guaranteed to last. They are usually given with aspirin or other pain-relievers.

These drugs which produce remissions were discovered to be useful purely by accident.

In the days before the new antibiotics became available for treating tuberculosis, gold injections were often used for that disease. They did not have much effect on the tuberculosis, but it was observed that when some patients with rheumatoid arthritis were treated (because at one time this disease was thought to be related to tuberculosis), the arthritis improved. Similarly, in the prevention of malaria in people going to the Tropics it was found that some of the drugs used also led to considerable improvement in arthritic patients. For these reasons, the use of these two types of drugs has been carefully tried out in patients with rheumatoid arthritis – and proved to be beneficial.

But that is where the good luck stopped! Although gold is effective there are undesirable side effects, particularly involving the skin, the kidneys and the blood. If the patient develops itching or any sort of rash, then it is essential that he tells the doctor and the gold injections are stopped. Because of this element of doubt, precautions are always taken: the urine is tested before each injection, the patient is given regular blood tests, and if he develops any sore throats or other ill-effects, then the gold is discontinued. Despite all this, gold remains one of the most effective treatments we have and, with strict precautions, should be safe.

The drugs discovered from treating malaria (chloroquine and hydroxy-chloroquine) also have their own unwanted effects. One of these relates to the eyes, so that regular eye check-ups by an ophthalmic surgeon are important. In a recent review, one hospital found that serious eye trouble caused by these drugs occurred only once in 7,000 patients – so it is not common.

There is another new drug called penicillamine which should be mentioned here. It is related to penicillin but is not itself an antibiotic. Quite how it works is not known but sometimes it is very effective. Regular blood and urine checks are essential as with gold.

(c) *Cortisone and other steroids*. These drugs have a dramatic – indeed, almost miraculous – effect in relieving the arthritis. Once a patient with rheumatoid arthritis starts taking either cortisone or its derivatives (prednisone, prednisolone and similar compounds), all the symptoms and signs of arthritis can disappear virtually overnight. The introduction of these drugs was accompanied, not surprisingly, by an enthusiastic belief that here at last was a cure for rheumatoid arthritis.

But sadly these hopes have not been sustained; the drugs are certainly very effective in the short term, but in the long term patients generally do as well or better without them. Moreover, they can also produce very severe side effects! The principal problems of these particular drugs are that they are liable to produce indigestion or ulcers in the stomach, and they can seriously weaken the bones and muscles. Also after a few months of treatment the face becomes red and rounded (moon face) and women may grow moustache hairs. Doctors therefore try to avoid their use whenever possible.

But sometimes it is not possible. They are so effective that in severe disease their immediate use may be required: nothing else will help. The dose is, however, reduced as soon as possible and restricted to the essential minimum. From time to time efforts are made to withdraw the drugs entirely. For long-term use these drugs are relatively safe if taken in very low doses. The temptation gradually to increase the amount must be strictly resisted.

Any patient who is receiving steroid preparations must carry a steroid identity card at all times. This is because dependency on steroids develops. Dangerous complications may follow if their use is suddenly stopped for any reason. The card contains details of the steroid preparation that the individual is taking – that is how much and for how long – together with his doctor's name, address and telephone number. If the patient should be run over by a bus, suffer from a heart attack, need an emergency operation, or anything else happens which makes him unable to give this information, the card will tell any medical person who is present that steroids are essential.

If the arthritis is generally under good control but one or two joints are inflamed and troublesome, it is sometimes possible to inject steroids directly into those sites. This will control those particular joints but is effective only for a few weeks. Repeated injections are not a good idea as in the end they may themselves damage the joint.

(d) *Drugs that suppress immunity.* It has recently been found that a special group of drugs will suppress the immunity mentioned at the beginning of this chapter and can be effective in patients with arthritis. However, their use is restricted to patients with very severe disease. They must be kept under close observation by a doctor and must have regular and frequent blood checks to make sure that the correct dose is not being exceeded.

Some remarkable improvements have occurred in patients who 'failed' on all other treatments, but these powerful drugs are definitely only indicated in very special circumstances.

(e) *Drugs to treat the complications of rheumatoid arthritis.* Many patients with rheumatoid arthritis are more ill than they need be, not because of the arthritis but because of one of its complications.

Anaemia is one of the commonest of these, usually due to iron deficiency, and is treated by iron pills or injections. Patients with severe disabilities are also liable to anaemia from poor nutrition. They have difficulty in getting food, or, having got it, in cooking and preparing it, especially if they live alone. There may then be other dietary deficiencies as well for which the treatment may of course be different.

(f) *Radio-active injections.* Recently minute amounts of a radio-active chemical known as Yttrium-90 have been used for injection directly into joints such as the knee. In the right circumstances it can be successful in controlling inflammation in that particular joint.

(g) *Research into drugs for rheumatoid arthritis.* One factor that has become clear from discussing the drugs currently in use for rheumatoid arthritis is that a sixth 'category' is needed to stress the need for research into new – and old – drugs.

Many new drugs are being developed for the treatment of rheumatoid arthritis. Some of these represent real advances and others only mimic the effects of preparations in current use. Research into drugs is essential. It is imperative to find out precisely how these drugs work. If it is possible to identify the ways in which they are helpful and to learn how to avoid the harmful effects, then it may be possible to design a successful new drug.

In clinical practice it can be difficult to decide whether a new drug is of real value, especially if it is presented in a brightly coloured form. The patient may 'believe' in it and feel that it must be doing some good, whilst even the doctors can be misled in a similar way. For this reason, trials of new drugs must be carefully designed and comparisons drawn with drugs of known value, so that the true worth of the preparations can be properly established.

6 Surgical treatment of rheumatoid arthritis

In the last few years rheumatologists have cooperated with orthopaedic surgeons to develop a combined approach in treating these patients. Many new operations are being performed and these have dramatically improved the outlook for patients with joint damage.

In the early stages of the arthritis the inflamed synovium or joint lining may be removed by the operation of 'synovectomy'. Similarly, if the sheath of a tendon is affected by the disease, then this inflamed synovium can also be removed.

Another situation which benefits from surgery is when a nerve is trapped by the inflamed and swollen tissue. A common site for this is at the wrist; here, the nerve passes through the front of the wrist to supply the index, middle and half the ring finger. The trapped nerve produces 'pins and needles' and a feeling of numbness in these fingers, together with pain in the hand and arm at night. Freeing this nerve by a very minor operation will immediately remove this symptom.

In advanced severe disease there have been some exciting

developments in the replacement of damaged joints by new spare part artificial joints. The most successful of these operations has been on the hip joint, where it can be expected that over ninety per cent of the replaced hips will function successfully. They should provide complete relief from pain and a good range of movement. New plastic joints are also now being used for the fingers; by correcting much of the deformity and allowing a better use of the hands, these are very effective. Replacing the knee is an operation which is still being developed; this can be very successful in some patients but it has not yet reached the same advanced stage as operations on the hip. There are also artificial shoulders, elbows and ankles which are available in some hospitals.

The outlook for rheumatoid patients

After this rather gloomy account, any arthritic readers must surely have been plunged into despair – or put the book away after the first few depressing sentences – and are perhaps anticipating severe crippling in their own particular case.

Nil desperandum! (Do not despair!) The majority of patients with early rheumatoid arthritis have a transient attack which will clear up completely. Many of these patients never have sufficient symptoms to take to their own doctor and of those that are seen by their general practitioner, only some are severe enough to be sent to a hospital.

And for those that are sent to hospital, here are the not-so-grim statistics: they are by far the worst cases, and yet of these patients, a quarter will have their disease clear up completely without any remaining disability. A further quarter will heal, leaving slight joint damage but not enough to interfere significantly with their working lives. Forty per cent will suffer continual disease activity, which means that they may expect to suffer recurrent pain and be on drugs to control the arthritis, but nevertheless they will not be incapacitated or bedridden. It is only ten per cent or less of these hospital patients who risk becoming severely crippled.

Clearly it would be very helpful in planning treatment if

doctors could know which patients are likely to be amongst the lucky ones in whom the disease will clear up and which will be the unlucky ones in whom it is likely to go on to cause further problems. More vigorous treatment could then be given to the latter group in the early stage. Today there are two new tests which can give some information in this regard although not sufficient to be absolutely definite. If a patient has a lot of rheumatoid arthritis factor in the blood, and especially if he belongs to the white cell group HLA DW4, then he is more liable to develop serious disease which will go on for a long time. Trials of treating such patients with strong drugs at the beginning of their illness are being performed.

One thing which also brightens the outlook for patients has already been mentioned at the beginning of this section: this is that a massive research programme is at present underway to try to determine the cause of arthritis.

Much research is being done into the mechanisms of immunity and how they become disturbed in rheumatoid arthritis. Other studies are being directed at the actual ways by which various types of deformity develop. Many mechanical factors are involved and an improved understanding of these will lead to a better approach towards medical and surgical treatment.

In writing a book of this nature, there is always the problem of there being a number of less common items that do not readily fall into any of the standard chapters. In order to be comprehensive, a hotch-potch chapter describing these various less common types of inflammatory arthritis and rheumatism is therefore included. Many of these conditions can affect the spine and have already been given a brief mention in Chapter 2.

Arthritis and psoriasis

Psoriasis is a curious but very common condition of the skin. Once seen it is easily recognized – it appears as patches of thickened red skin that have a strong tendency to flake. Commonly sited on the back of the elbow, the front of the knee, and in the scalp, psoriasis can also appear anywhere on the trunk or limbs. The precise cause of this disease, as with so many medical conditions, is a mystery. Studies of the skin itself, including parts of the skin not affected by the actual rash, have shown that there are significant abnormalities in the behaviour of the skin cells and also of the smallest capillary blood vessels which bring oxygen and other nutrients to the skin.

Psoriasis can start at any age and often begins in childhood. It occurs in several members of a family more often than would be expected by chance, so perhaps there is some inherited predisposition to it. Sometimes one meets families in which one member has psoriasis and another member has mild arthritis and yet another member has both. But the true nature of this inheritance – if that is what it is – is still unknown.

Rheumatoid arthritis coinciding with psoriasis
Confusion can arise because both rheumatoid arthritis and

psoriasis are common conditions so, by sheer coincidence alone, they must occasionally develop together. The symptoms and signs of the arthritis are then exactly the same as those in any other patient with rheumatoid arthritis (as described in Chapter 4).

Psoriatic arthropathy

Rheumatoid arthritis coinciding with psoriasis should not, however, be confused with the type of arthritis directly associated with psoriasis – so-called 'psoriatic arthropathy'. Despite certain superficial resemblances to rheumatoid arthritis, this condition is an entirely separate disease with important distinguishing features.

Psoriatic arthropathy can affect any joint, but in contrast with rheumatoid arthritis it often affects only one or two joints. The joint becomes inflamed causing pain and swelling which then limits movement. The joints near the tips of the finger (which are hardly ever affected in rheumatoid arthritis) are especially prone to inflammation. When these joints are inflamed the corresponding finger-nails also show direct damage due to the psoriasis. In its mildest form there is very tiny pitting spread randomly over the nail, which is only detected on very close examination, but later the nail becomes severely damaged and is seen to be thick and discoloured. The nail may even become partly separated from the tip of the finger by a thick white chalky material.

Psoriatic arthropathy can sometimes severely destroy a joint and the inflammatory process may eat away the bony surfaces. In general, however, the arthritis of psoriatic arthropathy is less severe than ordinary rheumatoid arthritis and patients do better in the long run!

Psoriasis and the spine

Involvement of the spine is another – but uncommon – type of arthritis associated with psoriasis. In its simplest form there is inflammation at the bottom of the spine around the sacroiliac joints. These, you may remember, are the same joints as are involved in ankylosing spondylitis. In Chapter 2 it was mentioned that spinal changes similar to ankylosing spondylitis may develop with psoriasis. The low back pain and stiffness which characterize inflammation of the sacroiliac joints are the first symptoms, but the arthritis may spread from these joints up the spine towards the neck. After the initial stage of inflammation the bony changes of ankylosing spondylitis may develop with similar results – back pain and back stiffness, sometimes to the point of rigidity. It can be impossible to distinguish psoriatic involvement of the spine from true ankylosing spondylitis. Moreover, these patients often have the same white cell type HLA B27 as is found in ankylosing spondylitis. So obviously individuals with this cell type who develop psoriasis are at greater risk of developing these spinal problems.

Psoriasis and gout
Finally a brief reference must be made to the fact that the abnormal biochemical changes in the skin may lead to excessive production of uric acid in the blood which consequently may produce gout. This is rare, but when it occurs, it leads to great confusion in deciding upon the cause of arthritis.

Reiter's syndrome

The tradition of naming places after the explorers who discovered them seems to have seeped into medical custom, where several names of diseases have been derived from the first ostensible 'discoverer' of the condition. Hans Reiter in 1916 described the case of a Prussian cavalry officer serving in the Balkans who developed acute arthritis together with inflammation of the eyes and a discharge from the penis. Since then the disease has been called 'Reiter's Disease' or 'Reiter's Syndrome', but in fact the true credit belongs to an Englishman – Sir Benjamin Brodie – who described the disease almost a hundred years earlier in 1818.

A type of VD?
Again, referring to Chapter 2, it has been suggested that there is a possible relationship between Reiter's syndrome and venereal disease. In this country many cases occur as a form of venereal

disease, but not all. Reiter's syndrome may also follow as a result of infective diarrhoea.

The disease is probably due to some sort of virus and is transmitted directly from one person to another. Outbreaks of Reiter's syndrome have been described aboard ships in circumstances suggesting this type of infection. It is far more common in men than women and usually starts in young adults, features which, in terms of our knowledge about trends in sexual promiscuity, would be consistent with such an association. Direct proof is, however, still lacking. There is an additional factor which makes certain individuals susceptible to this disease. This is the same HLA B27 white cell group which was described in Chapter 2 and which is almost always present in patients with the spinal condition ankylosing spondylitis. It may be that a different kind of infection determines whether the patient gets Reiter's syndrome or ankylosing spondylitis, or sometimes both.

The symptoms

The early symptoms are certainly suggestive of venereal disease. The discomfort of a burning pain on passing urine is made worse by the fact that this often becomes a more frequent need than normal although only small volumes of urine are passed on each occasion. The sufferer may have to get up several times during the night in order to relieve himself. There is also usually a small discharge from the penis.

Within a couple of weeks, inflammation develops in either one or both of the eyes – this is called 'conjunctivitis' – and shortly after this arthritis appears. The joints become swollen and very painful. It is often the joints in the feet and knees that are affected, but it can be elsewhere. Ulcers may appear, usually on the penis or inside the mouth. Finally, there is also a skin rash appearing at first on the soles of the feet and then perhaps on the rest of the body. Reiter's syndrome can, as this description implies, be a very unpleasant disease.

Treatment

Treatment is with antibiotics, pain-relieving drugs, physiotherapy and rest, and given these the condition usually settles down within a few weeks. It is unfortunate, however, that there is a tendency to relapse and something like one-third of all patients suffer recurrent trouble. This creates more of a problem than just 'nuisance value', for after many episodes of arthritis, deformities of the joint may appear. The feet may become badly affected and changes in the spine, similar to those of ankylosing spondylitis, may develop. Another interesting point is that the skin rash resembles some varieties of psoriasis.

Ulcerative colitis and Crohn's disease

Ulcerative colitis and Crohn's Disease are both conditions in which there is inflammation of the bowel, and both are diseases which sometimes have the additional affliction of being accompanied by forms of rheumatism.

The two conditions, however, do differ in many details from each other. To understand these differences, a point of clarification is perhaps needed: in its passage through the body, food which enters the stomach passes out through the duodenum into the small intestine and then into the large intestine before any waste materials are lost. Ulcerative colitis is characterized by persistent inflammation of the large intestine, producing recurrent and sometimes severe diarrhoea. Crohn's disease, on the other hand, more frequently involves the small intestine.

Similar types of rheumatism may complicate both conditions. Inflammatory arthritis may occur in either the limbs or the spine.

Arthritis in the limbs

The more common complication with ulcerative colitis and Crohn's Disease is arthritis of the limbs. This is usually in the knees but can sometimes also affect the feet or elsewhere. Again, it is the same story – the joints become swollen, inflamed and painful, and may be difficult to move. Fortunately, the arthritis is usually mild and clears up spontaneously within a few weeks, rarely leaving behind any permanent damage. Usually, the degree of inflammation of the joints corresponds with that in the intestine, so that when the bowel inflammation improves with treatment, then inflammation in the joints subsides.

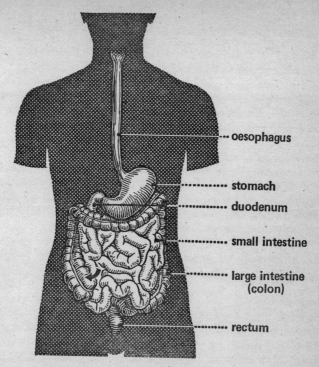

The digestive tract

Arthritis in the spine

Inflammation of the joints in the spine can also accompany these conditions, but this produces an entirely different form of rheumatism. Again, the sacroiliac joints at the lower end of the spine are affected first, with symptoms that are similar to those of ankylosing spondylitis; pain and stiffness in the low back is increased by resting and is especially bad during the night, whilst relief is gained through exercise. When the arthritis becomes more severe, inflammation spreads up the spine, revealing itself to be in fact, ankylosing spondylitis. The symptoms are precisely the same as described in Chapter 2 – stiffness of the whole spine is present and all movements become very limited. Eventually, the vertebrae can become jointed by bone so that all hope of further movement becomes lost.

Treatment lies in control of the bowel disease and prevention of stiffness by exercises and activity. Drugs such as aspirin or indomethacin are used to damp down inflammation in the joints.

These forms of rheumatism, although unusual, are of particular interest because they do throw some light on the causes of ankylosing spondylitis. Perhaps infection or inflammation in the pelvis can lead to chronic inflammation of the spine. There may be some underlying abnormality of the tissues leading to inflammation of the bowel and spine. And once again we also know that the same white cell tissue type HLA B27 is more common in the patients who develop spine inflammation.

Systemic lupus erythematosus and other auto-immune diseases

Immunity

There is a custom amongst many parents to encourage their children to 'catch' certain infections, such as German measles. This is, of course, no wild desire to nurse their child through these rather irritating conditions, but is an insurance against their contracting such diseases in future years. In other words, immunity to these particular conditions is encouraged because once a child has had German measles (or chickenpox, mumps, measles, and a host of other infections) he never gets it again. Furthermore, the disease in a child is usually less severe than in an adult.

The principles of immunization are quite simple although the details are extremely complicated. During the initial infection special proteins called 'antibodies' are produced by the tissues. These antibodies are directed at the particular invading organisms and eventually destroy them. Even after the disease has been wiped out the antibodies persist in the blood and therefore prevent further attacks. These antibodies can also be artificially stimulated in the body by appropriate injections so as to avoid an attack of a particular disease – as no doubt those of us who travel abroad are aware. These are the processes of vaccination and immunization as used for diphtheria, smallpox, measles, yellow fever, typhoid, and countless other diseases.

Auto-immunity

Antibodies therefore have a very important function in the body. They are there to protect us from infections. But occasionally things go wrong. Instead of antibodies being produced to fight

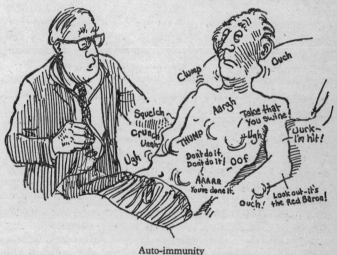

Auto-immunity

against invading bacteria or viruses they are developed against the body's own tissue. When this happens it is called auto-immunity.

Inflammation due to auto-immunity may occur in many structures in the body, including the joints, lungs, skin, heart, blood cells, kidneys and so on. This condition – when auto-immunity occurs attacking many parts of the body – is called by the rather complicated name 'systemic' or 'disseminated lupus erythematosus'.

Systemic lupus erythematosus

An understanding of the meaning of this name partly explains the characteristics of the disease:

systemic or disseminated – spread throughout the whole body

lupus – is derived from the Latin for 'wolf', which described the rash which may appear on the face. (It used to be thought to be similar to the effects of a wolf bite.)

erythematosus – from 'erythema' or redness, meaning inflammation occurring in the skin

Systemic lupus erythematosus is obviously a very complicated and unpleasant condition although, fortunately, modern drugs have done much to control it. It is included in this book because a prominent feature of the disease can be inflammation of the joints and rheumatism. Young women are most frequently affected and occasionally it follows the use of certain medicaments.

There is a wide variety of other related disorders (with equally fascinating names) which should be mentioned briefly:

In *Polyarteritis Nodosa* there is inflammation of the blood vessels. This may occur in many parts of the body but in particular may affect the blood vessels near joints and produce forms of arthritis.

Scleroderma is a peculiar condition in which there is considerable thickening of the skin. This is most marked in the hands, but may sometimes spread over other parts of the body. Because of this thickening the movements of the limbs, particularly of the hands, become very stiff and difficult.

Our understanding of this group of disorders is still limited. Research aimed at investigating the mechanisms of immunity and the disturbances in all these different forms of auto-immune disease is currently being carried out. Rheumatoid arthritis itself is closely related to this group of conditions, and a fuller understanding of one should aid in the understanding of all the others.

Venereal disease and arthritis

Reiter's syndrome has already been described as one form of venereal disease leading to joint disorders. It was presented earlier in the chapter because of its similarities to the arthritis relating to psoriasis and because Reiter's syndrome is not exclusively a result of venereal disease. Many instances follow dysentery.

Venereal diseases can cause a lot of troubles but the only ones with which we are concerned in this book are those accompanied by forms of arthritis.

Gonorrhoea

Gonorrhoea is the commonest form of venereal disease in this country and with the current relaxing of sexual morals particularly among the young, it has recently become extremely widespread. In fact, gonorrhoea is now the commonest single infectious disease in Britain! It is caused by a tiny rounded bacterium called the 'gonococcus', which is transmitted by sexual contact and infects the sexual organs. The major problem with gonorrhoea is that although the symptoms in men are obvious and painful, women who are affected often do not know it, so they fail to obtain proper medical treatment and continue to transmit the disease to their partners without ever realizing that they have it.

The onset of gonorrhoea is experienced as a burning pain whilst passing urine, usually with a discharge from the penis. A week or two later the sufferer may become generally ill with aches and pains in many joints due to a generalized infection of the body. Then eventually the infection may focus in one particular joint which becomes acutely inflamed.

Fortunately gonorrhoea usually responds successfully to penicillin, but it is most important that this treatment is started as quickly as possible.

Syphilis

Syphilis is a much more serious disease which has now become very rare. It is caused by a corkscrew-shaped bacterium different from the one described above and can in time produce terrible complications in many of the body tissues.

Many years after infection it can damage the nerves in the spinal cord that send the messages of pain from the legs to the brain. This has important results. With this loss of feeling of pain in the legs, the joints can be badly sprained without the person concerned being aware of any trouble at all. Normally, the pain from, say, a sprained ankle stops the sufferer from using it. It hurts too much and he has to rest it and with rest the damage rapidly heals. When, however, pain is absent, continual use of damaged and weakened joints may produce further damage and this is precisely what may happen in people who have had syphilis. Their joints suffer recurrent damage and eventually become destroyed. Despite being painless, the joints are unstable and easily 'give way', so preventing proper use of the limb. This condition is most frequently seen in the feet or knees which are then known as 'Charcot' joints, after a famous French physician who was interested in diseases of nerves.

These painless but damaged Charcot joints are not exclusive to syphilis – they are occasionally found in severe diabetes and in other diseases of the nerves. They sometimes develop (fortunately not in this country) in leprosy when the nerves are damaged by the leprosy bacillus.

6 Osteoarthrosis and wear and tear

The last two chapters have concentrated on inflammatory types of rheumatism; if, however, the doctor finds no evidence of inflammation in the bones and joints then the trouble is quite likely to be due to 'wear and tear'. This process of wearing out of joints has already been fully described in Chapter 1 in relation to the back (lumbar spondylosis) and in Chapter 3 in relation to the neck (cervical spondylosis).

A similar process of wearing out can occur in other joints where it is then called osteoarthrosis. This condition was previously, and perhaps more familiarly, called osteoarth*ritis*, but as the suffix 'itis' attached to any medical word is intended to reflect the presence of inflammation, the more apt name osteoarthrosis is correct. Although osteoarthrosis can affect many joints at the same time, it should not be regarded as a disease of the whole body like measles or rheumatoid arthritis. Each individual joint must be considered as an isolated problem.

Wear and tear – or ageing

Osteoarthrosis is a process which is inextricably related to the ageing of joints. It would be pleasant to believe that we are the same people throughout our lives, but the truth is that we are not. The supple young man of nineteen becomes the stiff old man of ninety with grey hair and a changed face. Similarly, changes also occur in the joints, bones, muscles, and tendons – all the things that can give rise to the various forms of rheumatism.

Many of these changes are painless: the fact that they happen so gradually tends to make them acceptable. It is only when the wearing process starts unusually early, causes pain or is exaggerated in any way, that it is called a 'disease'.

The question that must now be answered is – what exactly happens when the joints age? To understand this process, it is necessary first to comprehend the mechanics by which joints move.

Lubrication and repair

The human joint has a wonderful system of lubrication. Indeed, engineers would dearly love to be able to reproduce such a remarkable system, and have in fact learned of new principles of engineering by studying the living joint. The natural joint is more slippery than any simple engineering joint or bearing and only ball bearings and roller bearings create less friction.

How does this system of lubrication work?

1 the two surfaces have a high natural slipperiness. In this they resemble certain plastics which are 'self-lubricating', i.e., they provide their own lubricant;

2 the surface as revealed under the microscope is not smooth. It is pocketed in a series of minute undulations which trap joint fluid between the two moving parts;

3 the joint fluid is not an oil but a solution of mucus which under pressure 'loses' water and thickens up.

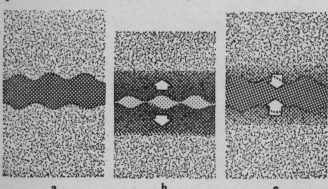

a   b   c

In the moving joint a film of mucus comes between the two surfaces where some of it gets trapped in the little pockets (a). Under pressure the fluid thickens and provides increased viscosity just where it is most needed (b). As soon as the pressure is removed from the surface, water is taken up and the joint fluid resumes its normal thickness (c).

This surface which forms the slippery end of the bone is called articular cartilage. It grows through childhood, after which it is then formed for life. If it is damaged, it has therefore only a limited power to heal. Partial healing will occur if, for example, a joint has been operated upon and some of the cartilage removed. Or if, when a bone breaks, the break extends down into the joint, again partial healing will occur.

Failure or fatigue

Having admired the joint as a remarkable engineering system, the time has now come to question the reasons for its occasional failures or, rather, less successful functioning.

Articular cartilage like any other substance, is subject to what the engineers call 'fatigue'. This means that after it has been compressed and released many times, it may pass the limit of its natural resilience and break down.

There are several explanations proffered to account for the cause of joints wearing out.

The first important theory suggests that joints wear out because of a failure in the lubrication procedures. There is, however, no acceptable evidence of this.

Another theory offered is that the surface is subject to minute abrasive wear which 'outpaces' its replacement.

The third, and probably most important, theory has suggested that the breakdown is the result of fatigue due to repeated impact shock. This relates to the bones as well as to the cartilage. The bones in the body have a certain elasticity. In jumping and running they absorb some of the force of the impact but when old bones stiffen, the 'elasticity' is less and the impact shock on the cartilage is therefore greater. The significance of this theory is in the practical implications for preventing osteoarthrosis. Exponents of such a theory would advise people to avoid being overweight (which increases forces of walking) and to use rubber heels on shoes, particularly when walking on hard pavements.

Ageing, however, is not the only factor which causes 'wear and tear'. Osteoarthrosis is often due to 'accelerated' breakdown. Although most human joints will last in reasonable working order for all of the traditional three score years and ten – and many even longer – there are certain 'predisposing factors' which encourage early breakdown.

1 The first is incongruity. This means that the two parts of a joint don't fit together as well as they should. Badly made joints of this sort seem to run in certain families. The lack of fit is a frequent cause of trouble in the hip joint. There are also conditions such as congenital dislocation of the hip (when babies are born with the ball of the hip joint out of its socket) and deformities of the joints after operation, which have much the same effect.

2 Sometimes the cause of an early joint breakdown can be attributed to chemical or biological changes. The commonest of these is when lime salts are deposited in the cartilage causing a condition which is called chondrocalcinosis. This is described in Chapter 7 in more detail. Inflammation damages the joint both by actually eroding some of the surfaces and by destroying the mucus which is responsible for the lubricating properties of the joint fluid. Even if the inflammation recovers the damage may have been such that the joint is liable to early breakdown later on.

The development of osteoarthrosis

The first minute changes of osteoarthrosis are visible even in childhood. The surface of the joint begins to break down in one or two places but the changes are microscopic and because the cartilage is so thick they do not affect the efficiency of the joint. However, by the twenties and thirties the cartilage changes increase so that they can be seen with the 'naked eye' and they progress until in the forties and fifties the affected joints begin occasionally to feel painful. Each joint responds to this by attempting to heal itself – sometimes with unfortunate consequences! The new cartilage which grows at the edge of the joint forms a hard knob which later becomes bony. These bony knobs (as you may remember from Chapter 1) are called osteophytes.

These knobbly irregularities at the edge of the joint are characteristic features of osteoarthrosis. It is these osteophytes which, by obstructing the joint as a hinge, prevent its normal range of movement.

Because each joint must be considered as an isolated problem, it is necessary to look at the way in which osteoarthrosis can affect each individual joint. These can be conveniently divided into the non-weight-bearing joints of the arms, and the joints of the legs that take the weight of the body.*

Osteoarthrosis in non-weight-bearing joints

The hands

Although many joints in the hand can be affected, there is a tendency for osteoarthrosis to appear mainly in the joints at the

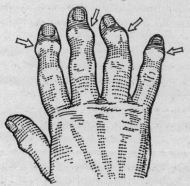

Heberden's nodes

ends of the fingers and the joint at the base of the thumb. Small knobs, at first soft but later bony, form on the backs of these joints.

This produces a characteristic appearance of the finger, and the bony prominences have been called after the physician who

* Wear and tear disease of the spine is entirely similar to that in the limb joints. It has already been fully described with reference to the low back and the neck in Chapters 1 and 3, respectively

first described them! But if calling these knobs 'Heberden's nodes' is a form of flattery or praise for William Heberden, then he deserved it: by describing this condition in 1803, Heberden stimulated scientific interest in the study of rheumatism. As a tribute to his work an important scientific society for research into arthritis has been named after him.

The pain in the finger when the Heberden's node is forming can be quite severe and often has a burning quality, worse at night. But usually the nodes are painless and cause little or no trouble. By contrast, osteoarthrosis of the thumb base joint is more often painful but since there is little to see (the joint is deeper inside the hand) it may not be immediately obvious that it too is forming a bony node.

Elbow, shoulder and jaw

The elbow and shoulder are seldom affected by osteoarthrosis. Virtually, the only times that they do become involved is after there has been some previous damage. Painful osteoarthrosis of the little joint at the top of the shoulder between the collar bone and shoulder blade, is, however, quite frequent, especially as a sporting injury. Surprisingly, the joints of the jaw just in front of the ear can be affected by the same problem and may on occasions make chewing painful.

Osteoarthrosis in weight-bearing joints

Knee

Arthrosis of the knee is very common. The knees creak and may make alarming grating noises, called crepitus, during movement. They become knobbly and may be difficult to straighten. The consequences are unfortunate – the subject is liable to be forced either into a 'bow-legged' or 'knock-kneed' position! The latter is more crippling because it is difficult to walk if the knees are continually colliding.

Operations for arthrosis of the knee are not as successful as in the hip and so are only performed as a last resort. However, this is a field of medicine where what is difficult today may be commonplace tomorrow.

Feet and ankles

The ankles are rarely affected by osteoarthrosis. However, the big toe joint, perhaps because of shoe pressure, is prone to the development of a bunion joint, known as hallux valgus. This is really a form of osteoarthrosis. Hallux valgus makes shoe-fitting very difficult. Further reference will be made to this in the chapter on feet – Chapter 10.

The hip

By far the greatest problem caused by osteoarthrosis is the damage and crippling, pain and misery it may cause to the hip. The hip is a fine example of a ball and socket joint, a joint which

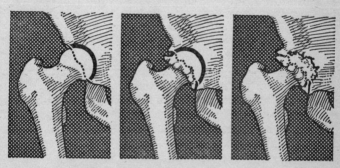

Stages in the development of osteoarthrosis of the hip

enables movement in any direction. But if the hip becomes affected by osteoarthrosis it gradually changes in shape as it wears down into a hinge joint which can only bend backwards and forwards. Characteristically, these patients cannot part their legs and in women this may make child-bearing or even sexual intercourse difficult or impossible by normal means. Only when the condition becomes really severe does it stop all movement in the joint.

Arthrosis of the hip is all too common – indeed it is one of the most frequent reasons why elderly people have to be cared for in long-stay hospitals instead of managing at home. Severe arthrosis of the hip causes a great deal of crippling for sufferers who, as a result, become frustrated and very restricted in their activities. For example, they may be unable to do such basic things as wash their feet, cut their toenails or put on stockings or socks without special aids. Walking more than about fifty yards may be excruciatingly painful. Even in bed there is no respite; a chance movement can, by causing pain, wake them at night.

Treatment

Operations for the hip

Twenty years ago in this country, and even today in other parts of the world, the fate of the patient with severe arthrosis of both hips was pitiable. Sufferers were in constant pain and virtually helpless; although operations might have relieved pain, they tended to leave the patient with an unpleasant limp.

One of the greatest revolutions in modern treatment of rheumatic diseases has been the development of special, 'spare part', hip operations known technically as total hip replacement arthroplasty. These were developed primarily by British surgeons and consist of artificial metal and plastic joints which are glued with special cement into the patients' own living bones.

When the operation is successful the artificial joint functions practically as well as a natural hip. For those who have been in pain for years a new hip can represent a new life.

How long will they last? Tests show that the artificial hip should last about fifteen or more years of vigorous life before it needs to be replaced, but for many old and frail patients, or those with trouble in other joints, the strain on the joint is likely to be less. In such cases the 'life' of the artificial joint will exceed that of the patient.

With modern anaesthetics the risks of the operation are small and it has been performed on patients over ninety (who would otherwise be helpless, bedridden cripples) as well as in children who would otherwise have no hope of a normal life. Most surgeons, in fact, have their patients up and walking between two and three weeks after the date of the operation.

As the modern operation in its present form has only been widely used for about ten years, the long-term risks are not yet

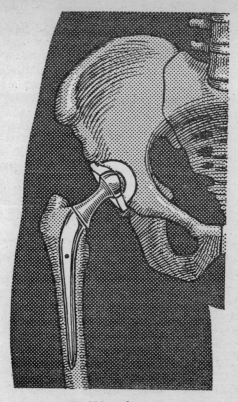

Total hip replacement

known though experimental work has been going on since 1955.
The over-all failure rate is surprisingly low, less than five per cent,
and this includes patients who are considered bad risk cases due
to other diseases.

Other methods of treatment

Aspirin may relieve the pain and stiffness of osteoarthrosis in
mild cases. The dose is important, however, as twelve or more
tablets a day may be needed to have an effect. Then there are
other standard pain-relieving drugs, including phenylbutazone

and indomethacin, which are particularly useful in the case of hip disease. But, as it was pointed out in Chapter 4, they all have their snags – in the form of undesirable side effects.

Warmth or heat administered in the same ways as recommended for other forms of rheumatism also help to alleviate pain. Many joints with arthrosis are cold-sensitive and need to be kept warm. So it is that a bandage around the knee, for example, probably provides relief through the warmth it supplies rather than for any other reason. The same effect can be achieved by using liniments that contain a warming chemical. Physiotherapists, as previously mentioned, have more sophisticated methods of providing heat such as short wave diathermy, infra-red machines and wax baths.

The question of rest or exercise is a controversial one. Usually, by the time a joint has become worn down and painful it is better

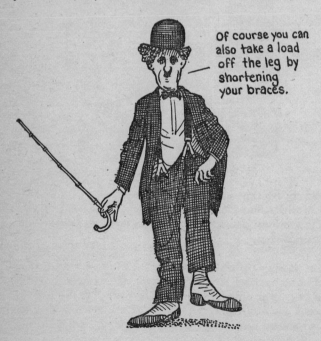

to 'keep it going' than to attempt to nurse it by continually resting it. If methods are used to alleviate the pain, it should not be too difficult for the sufferer to do some exercises. Swimming is useful, particularly when the hips and knees are affected. One traditional treatment is in the use of hot swimming pools which many hospitals and spas have available for rheumatism sufferers.

Local injections are used for the thumb base joint and for the small joint at the shoulder between the collar bone and the shoulder blade, with some success.

Trouble in the joints at the base of the toes may mean that shoes have to be purchased. Remember to have them fitted with rubber heels to absorb the shock of heel impact on the floor during walking. Remember also to use a walking stick, fitted with a modern non-skid rubber ferrule. It has been calculated that for a patient with osteoarthrosis of one hip, due to a leverage effect up to two-thirds of the weight can be taken off the joint by the use of a stick held in the opposite hand.

The future

Research is attempting to find methods of improving joint function and preventing fatigue failure. For example, both artificial and natural joint lubricants have been tried, but so far with only limited success.

Recently research workers have found that, even in 'ordinary' osteoarthrosis, one can find in the joints very minute crystals of the same material as is found in bone. Their research suggests that these crystals are not just made by wear and tear from the bone but are formed in the joint cartilage in such a way as to damage it and make it more easily liable to break down. This research is potentially helpful. If we can find a chemical (i.e. drug) that will stop these crystals forming then perhaps we will be able to prevent or treat osteoarthrosis more effectively in the future.

7 Gout and pseudo-gout

Gout is a 'snob' disease, more common amongst the rich, successful, aggressive and intelligent. Havelock Ellis studying all the people listed in Britain's *Dictionary of National Biography*, found that the famous names included had ten times the frequency of gout compared with people in the country as a whole. Gout's association with new-found affluence is vividly shown by the story of the Maoris in New Zealand, who, along with other Polynesian peoples, when they left their traditional fish and vegetable diet for the Western beef, bread, sugar and dairy products diet, showed an alarming tendency to overweight, coronary disease and, above all, to gout, which has now become something of a public health problem among them. Gout is also an ancient disease. One of the earliest written references to any particular illness is to gout. Hippocrates, the famous Greek physician of the fifth century BC, described the type of people likely to suffer from this disease with remarkable insight – even if the implications are somewhat tainted by the moral interpretations of his day.

'Eunuchs do not take the gout, nor become bald.'
'A woman does not take the gout unless her menses be stopped.'
'A young man does not take the gout until he indulges in coitus.'

Today the famous aphorisms of Hippocrates have to be taken with a pinch of salt. It is certainly true that gout is rare in eunuchs and in women; and when women do get gout it is usually after the menopause, but the third aphorism is much more likely to refer to Reiter's Syndrome (see Chapter 5) which in its post-venereal form frequently attacks the joints of the feet in young men in a manner resembling gout. Hippocrates' third aphorism is usually (and somewhat innocently) thought to mean that a boy does not get gout until after the age of puberty – which is broadly true although through modern experience gout is still fairly rare in men until the late thirties and forties. Surveys of primitive peoples living today have shown that Reiter's Syndrome is common amongst them. The Ancient Greeks were both medically primitive and socially promiscuous and even if intellectually advanced, they had no real way of telling one sort of acute arthritis (Reiter's) in the toes from another (gout).

The word 'gout' came from the Latin word 'gutta' meaning a drop. The theory – characteristic of the humoral theory of diseases at the time – was that drops of 'humours' would flow into a joint, and by distending it produce acute inflammation.

Inflammation due to crystals

Reasonable as these observations and theories seemed to be in the context of their age, we now have a more accurate and scientific knowledge of the conditions they were describing and of the relationship between gout and other diseases. True gout cannot exist without the deposition somewhere in the body, of the fine needle-like crystals of a compound of uric acid. These crystals are the signature of gout, so characteristic that if they are present in some material taken from the body when it is examined under the microscope, then the diagnosis *must* be gout, whatever else the patient is suffering. Most forms of rheumatism have nothing to do with crystals, but the lurid advertisement for bath salt 'cures' for rheumatism which used to show imaginary rheumatic joints packed with agonisingly sharp crystals have this element of truth in them – that one form of rheumatism, namely gout, has joints which can be filled with small sharp crystals. And although for most of the time these crystals are quite innocuous (individual crystals are only about the size of a red blood cell), on other occasions they can give rise to very serious pain. Some people with creaking joints think that the creaking and cracking means they have crystals in their joints – this is not so – the vast majority of noises coming out of a joint are due to other causes.

Crystals and crystalline structures are familiar to us all. Sugar, for example, is a very common crystal and in coffee sugar these crystals are grown to a large size so that it is possible to see that each has a definite shape by which it can be recognized. Common salt is also a crystal but it is ground sufficiently small for it to be almost impossible to spot the characteristic crystal shape of salt, although this can easily be recognized under a low-power microscope. Crystals which are known to cause gout and joint pain in man, however, are very small indeed and can only be seen with certainty under the highest power of the light microscope, whilst some (hydroxyapatite crystals – see the section on pseudo-gout) are so small that the crystalline structure can only be recognized by x-ray diffraction.

It is only in the last few years that doctors have realized that crystals can be responsible for other types of arthritis as well as for gout and these other types are listed under 'pseudo-gout'.

In the joint these tiny crystals can be engulfed by certain cells. Also within these cells, there are small bags called lysosomes which contain very powerful substances called enzymes. Enzymes are the factories of the cell, the means whereby it breaks down foreign substances which may penetrate its walls, and the means whereby (in tiny controlled amounts) it builds up the other substances needed for its life. Unfortunately these crystals are found by the cell to be indigestible. The lysosomes and their enzymes, instead of dissolving the crystals, are burst by the crystals with the result that the enzymes are liberated within the cell (which may die) and then into the joint, where they produce severe inflammation. The most well-known form of crystal-induced inflammation in the joint is ordinary gout. The particular inducing agent is crystals of uric acid, a relatively insoluble chemical which is deposited from the blood. The same type of acute inflammation can also be induced by other crystals.

Pseudo-gout, as its name suggests, resembles gout very closely, but is due to crystals of a different chemical derived from lime – calcium pyrophosphate.

Crystals and polarized light
How, therefore, do we discover and identify these crystals? The answer requires a basic understanding of polarized light pro-

cesses, since the only way to examine the joint fluid with certainty is by using the principle of the technique known as 'polarized light microscopy'.

Light travels in the form of waves and these waves vibrate in two directions – up and down and from side to side. In 'Polaroid' sunglasses a polarizing filter is used to allow light vibrating in

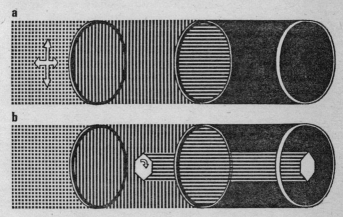

Recognition of crystals by polarized light

only one of these directions to pass through. The amount of light is cut by half. Two of these filters at right angles to one another will therefore not allow any light to pass. This is a simple experiment to test – look through two polaroid lenses, one in front of the other, then if one lens is slowly rotated, the view through both of them alternately disappears and reappears.

The relevance of gout to this interesting but apparently unrelated information is this. The recognition of the different types of crystals depends not only on their shape but on their ability to twist polarized light. When placed between two polarizing filters they will turn the light which has managed to pass the first filter and must be vibrating in, say, the up and down direction, into side to side vibration, so that it is then able to pass through the second. This enables the crystals to be seen brightly against a dark background. Joint fluid can be examined in this way and if crystals are found then the diagnosis of true gout or one of the forms of pseudo-gout can be made.

Gout – a gentleman's disease?

It is well known that gout is a disease of the well-to-do. The word itself elicits the image of the exquisitely dressed Regency gentleman quietly sipping his port, whilst the bottom of the picture shows an enormous bandaged foot.

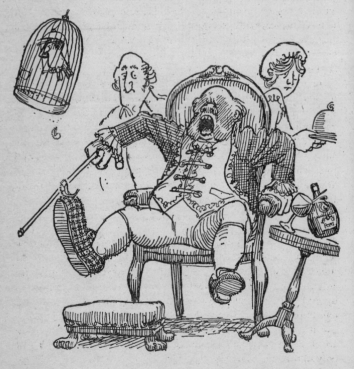

Special gout foot-stools used to be made, adjustable to the correct height, on which to rest the painful foot. They are now collectors' items.

Gout can affect any member of the population but certainly it is more frequent in the more affluent social classes. Its frequency is also related to degree of intelligence and for this reason, some students taking exams in the past have consumed vast quantities of uric acid in order to try to improve themselves. The results, however, were not quite those which were anticipated!

As Hippocrates said, gout is more common in men than women, and usually starts in young middle-aged males, whereas in women it only commences after about fifty years. Very, very rarely, true gout occurs in children. Certain forms of pseudo-gout (caused by crystals other than uric acid) are more frequent in teenagers.

Types of gout

True uric acid gout passes through two phases. Initially there is an acute stage, where the subject suffers from recurrent attacks of severe and often painful arthritis, almost invariably in the big toe joint. After each attack the toe seems to return completely to normal – until the next bout. But after a number of attacks, the stage of chronic gout is achieved; the joint gets progressively more damaged, it does not completely return to normal between attacks, but fluctuates between relatively painless deformity and relatively painful inflammation.

Acute gout

Of all the pains known to man, acute gout can be among the worst. In a bad attack, the joint becomes intensely swollen, inflamed and excruciatingly painful; it is so tender that the sufferer cannot bear even the slightest pressure to be placed upon it. The old joke says, 'If one of your friends took a large pair of pliers and squeezed the big toe joint hard – that's arthritis. But if one of your *enemies* did it, then that's gout.' By no means are all attacks as severe as this, but during a really bad attack, the only solution is to go to bed and rest. Even then the discomfort remains because of the often intolerable weight of the bedclothes.

Without treatment the attack usually lasts for a few days and then slowly improves.

Why is it that gout usually starts in the joint of the big toe? There is no fully proved explanation, but it seems likely that there are two main reasons. The first is that the big toe joint often shows osteoarthrosis (damage due to wear and tear) before all other joints, even in young people, and presumably because of the action of shoes. The second is that the big toe joint, being the joint furthest from the heart, is also the coldest joint in the body. These two factors, local damage – which is usually associated with local acidity of joint fluid – plus the lower temperature, both favour the crystallization of uric acid from its solution in the blood.

Chronic gout

Repeated attacks of acute gout eventually produce permanent damage because uric acid crystals sooner or later destroy the joint surfaces. The joint becomes filled with large masses of crystals looking like chalk. It appears very swollen and movements are limited and painful. It is also possible for an acute attack to occur where chronic joint damage already exists.

Gout tends mainly to damage the big toe joint, but destruction of the joints can also occur in the fingers, elbows and elsewhere.

Uric acid maybe deposited in other tissues. It is often found in skin on the backs of the elbows, on the margins of the ears and in the hands. Collections of uric acid crystals appear just beneath the surface and can sometimes burst through the skin producing ulcers which discharge their white chalky material.

Gout and the kidneys

The kidney is another part of the body which can be damaged by uric acid. Indeed, for practical purposes, it is the only internal organ of the body where gout can occur and fortunately even here it is uncommon. The condition is otherwise restricted to the joints and to deposits in the skin.

Kidney damage is probably more important in the long run than joint damage. Painful joints can make life miserable from time to time, but damaged kidneys threaten life itself, either directly because they fail to get rid of waste products, or indirectly because they lead to high blood pressure which in turn may lead to heart disease and stroke. Even when kidney damage is not too severe, it still has unfortunate results since uric acid itself is one of the waste products of the body and is normally got rid of by the kidneys into the urine (hence its name). If the kidney, damaged by gout, becomes even less efficient at getting rid of uric acid, then this makes the condition worse.

Uric acid

The problems of gout centre around the formation and removal of uric acid. If you make too much of it, or if you fail to get rid of it, then the waste accumulates in the body and the result, sooner or later, is gout.

It is by no means the case that all the uric acid in the body comes from the diet. Some is produced by the building up and breaking down that goes on within all the cells in the body – muscle cells, liver cells, blood cells; all are being continuously manufactured to replace worn-out cells. Biologists speak of this as cell turnover, much as a shopkeeper, stocking up his shelves and emptying them again, would talk about his turnover. Part of the uric acid in the body results from this normal cell turnover. But in certain blood conditions, such as polycythaemia (too many red cells) and in skin conditions, such as psoriasis, the amount of cell turnover is greatly increased; thus people with these diseases are particulary liable to gout.

Part of the uric acid in the body comes from the cells in the food we eat, and foods which contain a lot of cells are traditionally liable to bring on gout. The principal foods containing them are liver, kidneys, sweetbreads, brains, meat extracts, fish roes, anchovies, sardines and whitebait. However, this list is not exclusive.

The third way in which uric acid is manufactured in the body is by direct chemical synthesis, without being built up into the proteins of the cells. A man who eats no meat, fish or offal and therefore gets no cells as part of his food, but who gets all his protein in the form of cheese, will still make more uric acid in his body than a man existing on a purely vegetarian diet. So it is not just the type of food that matters, but also the amount of it.

So much for the ways in which uric acid is made in the body.

If any of these methods of manufacture is over working, gout may result. But gout may also be developed if the methods of manufacture are all working at normal speed, but the methods of getting rid of uric acid begin to fail. Some of the body's uric acid is disposed of in the skin and some by passing into the digestive juices in the bowel where it meets bacteria which are capable of breaking it down. Up to one third of the uric acid produced is eliminated in these ways.

But by far the largest amount of uric acid passes by a complicated route through the kidneys and is excreted in the urine. People with large quantities of uric acid in the body and who lose excessive amounts through the kidneys, may develop kidney stones and renal colic.

We have already seen how kidney damage can cause the kidneys to be less efficient at getting rid of uric acid, but it is not the only factor. People who drink alcohol 'burn it', just as sugar is 'burnt' in the body to provide energy. In this sense, alcohol is definitely a food and is indeed sometimes used by doctors (in small amounts) for patients who have difficulty in taking solid food. But alcohol is not just burnt as it would burn in a spirit lamp. In the body it passes through the stage of transformation to lactic acid. People who drink quantities of alcohol have a lot of lactic acid in their blood and lactic acid can affect the kidneys and so stop them getting rid of uric acid. The more alcohol, the less uric acid is eliminated. It is easy to see that people who eat well (producing more uric acid) and who drink well (disposing of less uric acid) are those who are liable to gout.

Aspirin (acetylsalicylic acid) is one of a number of slightly acid drugs which also have the power to influence the rate of elimination of uric acid, and this is why gouty people should not take aspirin for headaches. For them paracetamol is better. There are other important drugs used for other diseases which may interfere with the elimination of uric acid via the kidneys and therefore cause gout.

The other key to the understanding of the role of uric acid in gout is in its solubility. Uric acid circulates in the blood in the form of its poorly soluble salt, monosodium urate. If warm blood is shaken up with uric acid in a test tube, for example, the maximum amount that will dissolve is only about 6 mg in 100 ccs. But blood is traditionally thicker than water, and the 'thickness' is due to plasma proteins which are able to keep uric acid in solution to levels far above the natural solubility. Because of this, all gouty persons, unless they are on treatment, have more, and sometimes two to three times as much uric acid in the blood than is desirable because of simple solubility. In chemical terms, their blood is a 'super-saturated solution of uric acid', and as any chemist will tell you, a super-saturated solution is one which very easily can be made to deposit crystals.

So it is with uric acid crystals. In persons with gout there is a strong tendency to form crystals, and for local reasons the tendency is strongest in the joints and kidneys. As long as a super-saturated solution occurs, then so long will crystallization continue.

In the past, before there were any effective treatments, some unfortunate sufferers would accumulate as much as half a pound of solid uric acid on and about their bodies. Enormous white chalky lumps could be seen. Today, with effective treatments, most medical students in training will never see gout as bad as that – they will only read about it.

The solubility of uric acid in blood is also a clue to the cure of gout. If the amount of uric acid dissolved in the blood can be kept down below about 6 mg in 100 ccs, then crystals of uric acid will steadily dissolve back again into the blood. And as we will see later in this chapter, this can be made to happen.

Treatment

Eating

If gout is associated with 'rich' living, then treatment must surely imply that a rather more spartan lifestyle is needed. However, mainly because of the miracles of modern medicine, this is not so. There are certain protein foods – as listed on page 137 – which have a high content of cells and therefore have a high potential for forming uric acid in the body. It would seem wise to avoid eating them as far as possible. But in fact, the drug treatment of gout is now so effective that it is hardly necessary to impose severe dietary restrictions on patients, other than the commonsense one that if a person is obviously over-eating and over-drinking, he should bring this down to sensible levels. If the gout can be controlled without having to be a martyr to a special diet, so much the better.

... and drinking

It is valuable to drink plenty of fluid such as water, tea or coffee, etc. Five or six pints a day will increase the flow of urine considerably and will help prevent kidney damage or stones from appearing.

However, the above advice will not provide an excuse for the gouty subject to disappear to his 'local' every night, for the recommended five or six pints of fluid – alcohol is certainly not a part of the cure! Gout and alcohol are traditionally associated with each other and there is some justification for this. Publicans, hoteliers and brewery workers, for whom alcohol is an 'occupational hazard'; stockbrokers, bankers and commercial travellers, who are exposed to the necessity of frequent business lunches; and others who live well such as businessmen and, let it be admitted, doctors, all have occupations whose members have more gout than other more abstemious people.

But alcohol is not related to gout only because of lactic acid affecting the kidneys. In the days before there was proper control of pollution, lead workers were especially liable to gout due to lead damaging the kidneys. Even today, people who distill illicit 'moonshine' whisky in the United States get very severe gout, not because of the alcohol, but because of the lead in it due to contamination from old lead piping, solder in old car radiators, etc, from which they make their 'do-it-yourself' stills.

There is one other way in which alcoholic drinks can affect gout. Some people, already gouty, find themselves sensitive to certain types of wine. For them champagne, perhaps, or port, can regularly bring on an attack, when a whisky and water, containing the same amount of alcohol, would have no such effect. Port in particular has a specially bad reputation for producing acute attacks, but other wines may equally be responsible.

So, as with all other things in life, it seems that moderation in drinking alcohol seems to be the correct advice!

Treating the acute attack

Gout is one of those diseases that seems to have suffered from an old precept that the more a treatment hurts, the more good it is doing. In the past, acute gout was so painful that extreme types of treatment were performed in order to relieve the symptoms. Unfortunately these methods were not based upon an accurate knowledge of the disease; terrifying 'cures' such as scarifying the joint with a knife, applying burning compresses, or blistering the skin over the joint were common. Indeed the treatment was often worse than the disease. But because an acute attack of gout usually only lasts two or three days the subsequent relief was seen as evidence of the value of the treatment.

Today treatment is rather more civilized as well as more effective! The most common drugs used are colchicine, indomethacin and phenylbutazone. When taken in correct amounts they will relieve the severe pain in only a few hours.

Colchicine is a drug with an interesting history. The Byzantine physicians in Constantinople discovered that a particular substance extracted from the autumn crocus provided an effective form of treatment. It was subsequently used in Europe up to about the thirteenth century, when somehow colchicine became lost to medicine. It was not rediscovered until the late eighteenth century, and it was the gout sufferer Benjamin Franklin who is credited with the introduction of the drug in America. Colchicine is still responsible for providing relief to many patients with gout but it is tending to become obsolete since modern drugs are equally or more effective and on the whole their adverse effects are less troublesome.

Gout and aspirin, however, do not mix. Aspirin in all its forms and in the proprietary mixtures which may be purchased at the chemist, is to be avoided in treating gout. This is because aspirin affects the complicated pathways by which uric acid is lost from the body through the kidneys. Instead of helping the situation it may do the exact opposite, by actually reducing the loss of uric acid from the body.

Advising a person suffering from a severe attack of gout to rest is like telling a man without legs not to walk. The joint is so painful that the subject is not capable of anything but resting. People with milder attacks, however, need this advice because walking around will usually make them worse. When the big toe joint is affected, resting in bed can only be effective if the foot is protected from the weight of the bed clothes. A specially designed hospital cradle will lift the clothes off the foot, but if this is not available, a large cardboard box with two sides cut out of it will suffice.

Treating chronic gout

The drugs used for acute gout (colchicine, indomethacin and phenylbutazone) do nothing to reduce the amount of uric acid in the body. Although they relieve gout's pain, they will not prevent further attacks nor will they alter any uric acid deposits in the skin, joints or kidneys.

However, in recent years, a fuller understanding of the complicated pathway by which uric acid is formed and removed has led to the development of effective drugs designed to reduce the amount of uric acid in the body. These drugs are of two types:

1 drugs which reduce the formation of uric acid, such as allopurinol;

2 drugs which increase the loss of uric acid through the kidney, such as probenicid.

Once it is necessary to start taking these drugs, it is almost always essential to continue the treatment throughout life. To put it simply, if bluntly, 'treatment for gout is treatment for life'. Fresh attacks of gout will be prevented and the joint swellings, the damage to joints seen on x-ray, and the visible deposits of uric acid in the skin will heal.

Unfortunately, during the first few weeks of treatment these drugs may actually stir up the gout. The reason for this is not at all clear, but it seems that they exert such a profound influence in removing uric acid from the deposits, where it is relatively harmless, that 'free' uric acid becomes available and gets into new, sensitive areas. There is a danger here which a patient does not readily understand. If he takes a drug for gout and it seems to make his gout worse, why should he persist? Obviously he won't think much of the new treatment unless the problem is explained to him and he is warned in advance. However, this is a problem which need not dismay those who want a 'long-term' cure from gout; these initial painful attacks can be prevented by taking small doses of the acute attack drugs during the first couple of months of treatment with the chronic gout drugs.

Today, gout should be completely controlled and the motto should be 'there can be no excuse for gout'.

Research into gout

Gout is perhaps the best example in rheumatology of how research can lead to effective control of a disease. Improved understanding of the complex way in which uric acid is formed and lost from the body has led to the development of specific drugs and to the present satisfactory situation. Nevertheless, knowledge is never complete and there is still a lot more work in progress aimed at pinpointing the various biochemical problems which initiate gout, and at defining specific abnormalities to enable us to have an even better understanding of the disease.

Pseudo-gout – chondrocalcinosis

Uric acid is not the only crystalline substance that can produce acute joint inflammation. For many years doctors have recognized that there is a special form of arthritis due to chalk-like substances other than uric acid being deposited in the joints. This material was later discovered to be a crystalline form of a substance derived from lime – calcium pyrophosphate. The similarities of the inflammation induced by this chemical to that induced by uric acid is reflected in one of its names – 'pseudo-gout'. It is also called 'calcium gout' and another name, which is perhaps rather more difficult to remember, is 'chondrocalcinosis'. The reason for this second name – 'chondro' refers to the cartilage and 'calcinosis' means calcium.

Chondrocalcinosis can affect adults at almost any stage, the only distinctive feature being that it sometimes runs in families.

Characteristically, it is the knee joint which is affected by this condition but it can also occur elsewhere, such as the wrist, elbow, hip, shoulder or spine. The trouble usually becomes apparent because of repeated attacks of severe arthritis, which can be as painful as in acute gout. Sometimes, however, the condition produces chronic wear and tear – or osteoarthrosis – and then the symptoms take the form of aches and pains and a feeling of 'grating' in the joint.

It is the x-ray that provides the clue to the diagnosis. This shows the abnormal chalky material and leads the doctor to examine some of the joint fluid under the polarizing microscope. The particular crystals of calcium pyrophosphate will then be discovered.

Chondrocalcinosis, although no one really knows why, sometimes coincides with other diseases. Unfortunately, treatment of these diseases does not relieve the arthritis.

Treatment
Aspirin, indomethacin, phenylbutazone and other similar drugs are usually effective, severe pain subsiding within one or two days. It may be helpful to take small amounts of these drugs continuously to prevent any relapse.

Research
Calcium pyrophosphate is formed in excess quantities by the cartilage cells in this disorder. Moreover it is destroyed by a particular enzyme which is missing in this condition. The result is that calcium pyrophosphate accumulates and is deposited in the joint. In the future if we can devise a method of replacing this enzyme then it should be possible to cure this condition.

Calcific periarthritis

Calcific periarthritis is another form of crystal gout in which a different chemical – calcium hydroxyapatite – is involved. In contrast with pseudo-gout, this substance is deposited in the soft tissues around the joint, but not actually in the joint lining. Inflammation is produced in precisely the same way. Whereas chondrocalcinosis affects old people and sufferers are usually in their sixties and seventies and more, calcific periarthritis is more often seen in young adults, and occasionally even in children.

8 Soft tissue rheumatism

In a book of this nature, one would assume that the most relevant or rather, the more interesting information would perhaps be about those numerous rather minor, but nevertheless painful conditions that most of us suffer from at various times in our lives. Few people visit the doctor to complain of having a stiff neck, a stitch or cramp, nor do they feel it necessary to see him because of aches and pains which they know by experience will disappear when they are less tense or perhaps when the cold winter is over. So, whilst the other conditions so far described in this book will have been explained – if only briefly – to the patients by their doctors, most of us remain in ignorance about these more general, less serious conditions.

This chapter will therefore deal, in some detail, with many of these soft tissue types of rheumatism.

The distinction between soft tissue and hard tissue is this; rheumatism in hard tissues refers to the various well-known, well-defined, and sometimes serious causes of arthritis which arise in the joints and bones of the limbs and spine (such as described in the previous chapters). Soft tissue rheumatism refers to a very large group of miscellaneous and ill-defined painful conditions which seem to arise in the fleshy parts.

Therefore, although none of the conditions about to be described in this chapter necessarily relate to each other (that is, if you have one kind of soft tissue rheumatism, it does not necessarily mean that you are liable to get the others), they do have one common feature which is that they all seem to arise in the 'soft tissues' of the body.

The extent of the problem

These particular types of 'aches and pains' are indisputably common. The latest figures show that soft tissue rheumatism of one sort or another causes a loss of 10 million work days to industry and each individual worker affected loses an average of twenty-two days per man or woman. Ironic as it may sound, if one considers this staggering total in relation to the number of days lost each year to industrial disputes, rheumatic illnesses of this type represent as large a problem to the economy as do labour strikes. And, enormous as the total is, it certainly does not justly represent the frequency of these conditions, since many of the sufferers continue to work and others are housewives and retired people. The problem is so common that everyone gets soft tissue rheumatism in one form or another at some time in their lives. Some forms, like cramp and stitch, are universal, mild and hardly disabling. Other kinds are serious and quite crippling.

There are two types of soft tissue rheumatism:

1 'Generalized', that is, affecting many parts of the body.
2 'Localized', which means arising in one or two areas only.

Generalized soft tissue rheumatism

These conditions affect people who 'ache all over' or who after resting seem to stiffen up so much that they feel pain when attempting to move about again.

Doctors who deal with rheumatic conditions have to be on their guard with this type of complaint, since as we know by experience, generalized aching is sometimes the way in which non-rheumatic diseases begin. Influenza, as an obvious example, often begins as aching in the neck, shoulders and back. Even some kinds of cancer affecting the bones occasionally start in this way. However, blood tests and x-rays (or just a few days of observation) will usually enable the doctor to give a clear diagnosis.

Fibrositis

Fibrositis, as you may remember, has already been briefly referred to in Chapter 1 as 'non-specific back pain', and in Chapter 3 as a cervical fibrositis, where a general ignorance as to its exact cause was confessed.

The word itself – fibrositis – is no longer a medical term

despite its official sounding name. It refers to aching and tenderness in the muscles, particularly those at the back of the neck and head, and in the soft parts at the top of the shoulder. It is also sometimes used with reference to a similar type of aching where the muscles of the low back join the pelvis.

Although fibrositis is extremely common, particularly in the neck, people vary tremendously in terms of how frequently they suffer from it and the type of conditions that initiate it. Certain factors tend to aggravate the pain for particular people: some people only suffer from it when they are ill, tense, tired or worried, others when they are chilled or have been in a draught. Some people only get it whilst they are incubating a cold, and some unfortunate people suffer all the time. One of the commonest causes is sleeping soundly with the head and neck in an awkward position because of the height of the pillows. Children seldom suffer from this because of the suppleness of their necks but it is particularly important for old people to have a pillow which is exactly right to allow for the stiffness of their necks.

Fibrositis is not a disabling condition and is in fact rarely more than a recurrent nuisance. If it does become more prolonged and incapacitating then more intense treatment is required. Temporary relief of fibrositis is gained either by rubbing the painful area or by applying heat or liniments that contain something which generates a feeling of warmth. However, Chapter 3 has already dealt extensively with the treatment of the painful neck.

One warning worth mentioning though is about frequent massage. What happens is that massage provides temporary relief, but much of the deep massage, which is given sometimes very forcibly, bruises the muscles. Not surprisingly therefore, the trouble is now heightened, the patient returns the following day requiring more massage – and so the story goes on!

Polymyalgia rheumatica
A disease of the elderly, and sometimes of the not so elderly.

Polymyalgia rheumatica is one of the commonest causes of generalized soft tissue rheumatism after the age of sixty-five. As a cause of rheumatism, it is at least as common as gout and affects about one in every two hundred people of that age group.

The onset of this disease is often quite sudden, affecting older people who up till then have been remarkably fit and vigorous for their age. The sufferer feels generally ill and feels pain in the neck, back, shoulders and thighs, though thankfully not all at the same time. The striking characteristic of this condition is the way in which the afflicted person stiffens up after resting. This is particularly bad in the mornings; in fact it is sometimes so severe that he is literally paralysed for an hour or more until the stiffening eases up.

A middle-aged person who gets polymyalgia rheumatica usually feels that he has become prematurely old; an old person often thinks his life is at an end. However, treatment in most cases is ridiculously simple. A few tablets of prednisolone produce an apparently miraculous cure after only a few days or even sometimes after a few hours. This particular drug was discussed in Chapter 4, where it was pointed out that prednisolone – a derivative of cortisone – is not without dangers. This source of 'a new lease of life' must only be taken under medical supervision and according to the results of regular blood tests.

The cause of polymyalgia rheumatica is unknown. It is not a disease of the muscles even though that is where the pain is felt. Sometimes it is associated with a disease in the arteries called temporal arteritis; this is a potentially serious condition which (by blocking vital arteries in the eye or head) can lead to blindness or a stroke. Again prednisolone acts as a 'magical' drug in preventing this.

A similar but extremely rare condition in younger people is caused by direct inflammation of the muscles and is called Polymyositis. The similarity is only in the symptoms – weakness, stiffness and a general tenderness of the muscles.

Other causes of generalized soft tissue rheumatism
There are many other types and causes of soft tissue rheumatism. The following list shows some of the strange assortment of factors that can cause this generalized aching and pain.

1 The commonest cause perhaps is the aching and tenderness in

the back and the limbs which some people get when they put on weight rapidly.

2 Older women who become 'hooked' on barbiturate sleeping tablets sometimes develop generalized aching.

3 Some younger women get similar aching when they take the contraceptive pill.

4 Veterinary surgeons who deal with cattle get a generalized form of rheumatism from sensitization to brucellosis (an infection in cattle) to which they are often exposed.

5 The neurological disease, known as Parkinsonism, may start in this way. Here the stiffness of movement is due to a disorder in the nerve control of the muscles.

Localized soft tissue rheumatism

'Localized soft tissue rheumatism' is a convenient term for grouping all the different pains, strains and aches that arise and are felt in a specific area due to a particular type of damage or strain on a part of the soft tissue.

The types of soft tissue rheumatism that will now be explained can be divided into groups according to the particular tissue affected.

1 Strained or sprained ligaments.
2 Tensed muscles.
3 Damage to the acromioclavicular or shoulder joint.
4 Inflammation or damage to the bursa (bursitis).
5 Swelling of the carpal tunnel in the wrist.
6 Swelling of the tendons (tendinitis).
7 Damage to the enthesis (tennis elbow, etc).

Strains and sprains
Strain occurs when a ligament is stretched. The ligaments, or check straps, work to limit movement in a joint. Therefore, if a joint is forced in a direction that it cannot bend, the particular ligaments stopping this 'impossible' movement become stretched.

An example will perhaps clarify this process: a person who

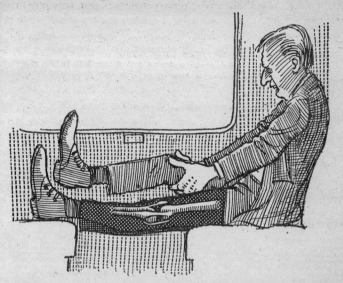

goes to sleep in a railway carriage with his feet up on the opposite seat will awake to find that his knees feel stiff and painful. This is because the whole weight of his leg has been hanging on the ligaments at the back of the knee, and it is only these, not his muscles, which have prevented the joint from bending back to front. These ligaments have been strained. Similarly, the gardener who is weeding a garden is 'hanging on his back' all day, and so may strain ligaments in his back. A patient who has suffered a stroke so that one arm is paralysed, will often experience severe pain in the shoulder joint because the whole weight of the paralysed arm is hanging on the joint without any protection by the muscles.

A Sprain, on the other hand, is a torn ligament. The most familiar example is the sprained ankle and the most common way of doing it is to run downstairs, miss one's footing and land so as forcibly to twist the foot inwards. The ligament at the outer side of the ankle, which is meant to stop it bending that way, gets torn. With such a tear, there may be bleeding and bruising under the skin. It is very difficult, even for a doctor, to know if it is the ligament which is torn (a sprain), or if a piece of bone to which it is connected has broken off (a fracture), without an x-ray. So unless there is only trivial pain, and particularly if there is a lot of bruising, the sufferer should always go to a hospital for an x-ray as soon as possible.

Tension headaches and neck pains

Most of the muscles in the body relax completely when they are not being used. But some muscles, known as the 'antigravity muscles' must work all the time in order to keep the body upright. For example, the jaw muscles must never relax, for if they did the mouth would fall open (as it does when a person falls asleep whilst sitting in a chair). Similarly, the muscles at the back of the neck must always be tensed otherwise the head would fall forwards when a person was sitting or standing.

Tension Headaches are often part of the problem of fibrositis. When people are worried they often tighten their muscles more than is necessary to hold the head upright. In other words, they are literally 'tense' and this in turn generates a strain on the places where the muscles are attached to the back of the head. The muscle attachments become tender and painful and when the pain is severe it will spread from the back of the head and neck, upwards and forwards over the head until it seems to be behind the eyes.

These tension headaches are very common and are often – wrongly – called 'migraine' by patients. The answer to them is usually quite simple: take a painkiller such as aspirin – a small dose of this will suffice – and get into a warm bed. A few minutes' sleep will allow the antigravity muscles at the back of the neck to relax and, miraculously, the headache will normally disappear.

A *Stiff Neck* is another common form of soft tissue rheumatism which is usually generated by tensed muscles. The muscles involved are again at the back of the neck, but are lower down than those which cause tension headaches. It is often associated with some change in the discs of the neck. Sometimes it is

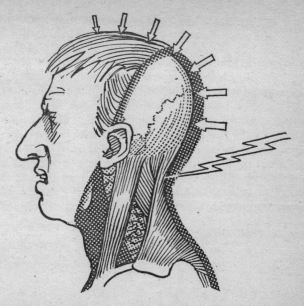

brought on by chilling or perhaps by sleeping on the wrong size of pillow.

The more severe causes of a painful neck have been described in Chapter 3. However, a word of caution is necessary here because a 'simple' stiff neck in a child or young adult may be an indication of something more serious. For example, a sore throat or mumps in a child may start as a stiffness of the neck, the stiffening in this case being due to swelling and pain in the glands of the neck. There will usually be fever as well. More sinister causes of a stiff neck in childhood are meningitis and 'polio', where the stiffness is due to inflammation of the spinal cord rather than the neck muscles.

In young adults, there is a particular form of stiffness called 'wry neck' or torticollis; in this condition there is a spasm of muscle such that the neck is not only stiff but the head is always being pulled to one side. Treatment can take a long time and, as the cause is not known, the condition is not easily curable and can be quite disabling. The unfortunate sufferer often notices that the neck spasm and twisting is worse when any work is attempted.

The painful shoulder*

Shoulder pains are common – ironically however, most of these pains come from the neck. There is a simple distinction between true shoulder pain and pain felt in the shoulder but actually arising from the neck; if it is difficult or painful to *move* the shoulder joint, then the trouble is arising from the shoulder – an obvious fact which is rarely appreciated!

Painful shoulders are sometimes due to trouble in the acromioclavicular joint – a little joint which connects the collar bone to the shoulder blade. Damage to this joint is a common sports injury but can often be rapidly relieved by injection treatment.

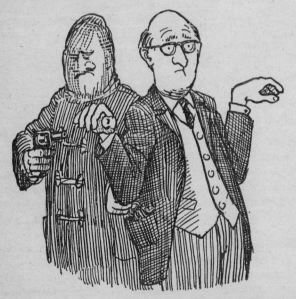

* Not included in this category is the stiff painful shoulders from which elderly people suffer caused by polymyalgia rheumatica. A blood test will indicate whether this is so, or whether it is purely a shoulder joint problem

Another type of shoulder pain is due to a peculiar condition called capsulitis of the shoulder. The popular name for this is 'frozen shoulder'. It affects people in the forty to sixty age range and often results in very painful, disturbed sleep. It is impossible, not just painful, for the sufferer to raise his arm high. The frustrations are obvious – women cannot even peg clothes on the line, and men find that they cannot reach things from a high shelf. 'Frozen shoulder' may take many months to get better, and often requires an injection, physiotherapy or manipulation under an anaesthetic.

But by far the commonest painful condition of the shoulder is 'bursitis of the shoulder' – a form of soft tissue rheumatism. This will be dealt with in the next category with the other conditions that develop as a result of some types of trouble with a bursa.

Bursitis

The bursa is the medical name for the space between a soft part of the body, usually a tendon or muscle, where it rubs over a bone or joint. The purpose is to lubricate this gliding surface (and so improve the efficiency of the body as a machine). But, like all machines, it can go wrong. A bursa can become rough or inflamed or even fill with fluid. It has a lining which is similar to that of a joint so it can also be affected in joint diseases such as rheumatoid arthritis or gout.

Bursitis of the shoulder

Bursitis of the shoulder is due to an inflammation of the tunnel through which the tendons that move the shoulder joint pass. The onset of this condition tends to be after the age of forty in most patients. The characteristic feature is that, although it is possible to raise the hand high above the head, as the arm is dropped downwards and sideways, pain develops over the 'middle range of movement' and then disappears when the arm is allowed to fall to the side. It is not difficult therefore to understand why this condition is often called 'painful arc'. Happily, however, it can often be rapidly relieved by injection treatment.

Housemaid's knee, beat elbow

These may sound a strange collection of medical names but the

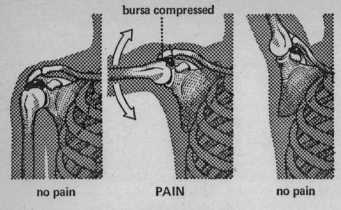

bursa compressed

no pain　　　PAIN　　　no pain

The painful arc

inference of each is fairly obvious, if not explanatory.

In Housemaid's knee, the bursa affected is the one which allows the skin to glide over the knee cap whilst a person is kneeling. Continuous pressure often causes it to become inflamed; this naturally affected housemaids who had to scrub the floors in the old-fashioned method by kneeling on the floor and scrubbing with a brush. Similarly it would affect nuns, or miners before the days of automatic coal-cutting machinery, when it was a common industrial injury known as beat knee. Beat elbow is a similar form of bursitis affecting the point of the elbow.

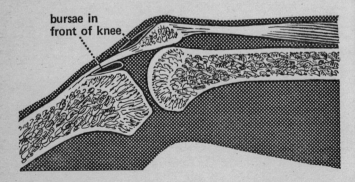

bursae in
front of knee

Bunion

A bunion is a painful swelling in the bursa which allows the skin to glide over the joint at the base of the big toe. It usually swells because of shoe pressures and is often made worse by bony enlargement or displacement of the underlying joint. A similar swelling over the base of the little toe is known as a bunionette*.

Snapping shoulder and snapping hip

These are conditions which, amazingly, often start as a type of party trick, but then become a habit. In 'snapping shoulder' the person finds that he can make a loud snapping noise by hunching his shoulder blade in a certain way. The noise arises from underneath the shoulder blade where it rubs over the muscles and ribs. However, there is a bursa in this spot which eventually becomes inflamed and painful. Snapping the shoulder seems to relieve the pain temporarily, but only perpetuates the condition.

In 'snapping hip' the trouble is similar but the snapping there is caused by a flat tendon which slips over the prominence of the hip during walking.

Carpal tunnel syndrome

When you clench your hand you can see a number of tendons passing from the muscles in the arms to the fingers; the tunnel through which they pass between the bones in front of the wrist is called the carpal tunnel. The lining of this is similar to a bursa and like the bursa may become inflamed and swollen. The problem of this swelling is increased by the fact that an important nerve – the median nerve – passes through this same tunnel to the hand and there is no room to spare. The swelling therefore immediately places pressure on this nerve and if the pressure is great, the nerve cannot conduct messages so that the index, middle and half of the ring finger will become numb. Pressure is seldom bad enough to block this nerve altogether, but it does cause irritation and severe pain. Characteristically, the pain, which has a special burning quality, spreads throughout the hand and arm when the pressure is severe. It is usually much worse at night and sufferers often describe how they hang their hands outside the bedclothes in an attempt to get some relief by cooling them.

* See Chapter 10 for information about rheumatism of the foot

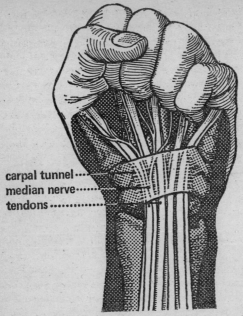

carpal tunnel ····
median nerve······
tendons ·············

The carpal tunnel

Carpal tunnel syndrome is quite frequent in early rheumatoid
arthritis but most examples have nothing to do with any generalized form of rheumatism. They came on because of gradual
thickening of the soft tissue in the front of the tunnel at the
wrist as the subject gets older. Most frequently affected are
middle-aged women and the problem is particularly common at
the change of life. However, it also occurs in men from time to
time and is a well-known complication of younger women when
they are pregnant. Relief can usually be obtained by a wrist
splint or by injecting a little hydrocortisone into the tunnel, but
some patients will require a minor operation to take the pressure
off the sensitive nerve.

Tendinitis
The tendon is the string or leader which connects a muscle to a

bone. Painful inflammation in the tendon is known as tendinitis, and a common area for this is on the thumb side of the wrist where one of the thumb tendons winds round the forearm bone. Another common place is at the back of the heel where the powerful calf muscles are attached. Inside the hand the swelling of a tendon or a lump forming on it, may give rise to 'Trigger finger'. The lump will not slide past a constriction in its tunnel. This condition – as reflected in its name – is manifested to the sufferer when he notices that the finger can be bent but then won't straighten unless actively pushed back with the other hand, when it then straightens with a snap.

Enthesitis

The enthesis is the place where the muscle is joined onto a bone; it is also the area in which the pain nerve fibres are particularly frequent.

The generalized stiffness and pain which affects people who are out of training and have been doing some hard exercise is probably due to minor damage to the entheses. But there are two or three specific forms of enthesitis that are very common and persistent causes of soft tissue rheumatism:

Tennis elbow arises where the powerful forearm muscles join the bone at the outer side of the elbow. *Golfer's elbow* is similar but affects the inner side of the elbow.

Policeman's heel is again a similar condition, but exists beneath the heel. The *Pelvis* is also sometimes affected where some other powerful leg muscles are joined to the bone.

Inflammation of many entheses occurs in ankylosing spondylitis (Chapter 2) in different sites in the body.

Treatment

Almost all local causes of soft tissue rheumatism are treated by local injections of cortisone with or without a local anaesthetic. It is often very effective and sometimes one injection only can produce a cure. For difficult or recurrent problems, long-acting derivatives of hydrocortisone are available. Occasionally minor operations are needed.

The likes and dislikes of rheumatism!

There are certain conditions and factors which seem to increase the occurrence and frequency of soft tissue rheumatism. Cold-sensitivity, poor blood supply and over-supple joints can make people particularly liable to suffer from certain rheumatic conditions.

Cold-sensitive rheumatism

Many rheumatic conditions are cold-sensitive, that is the pain seems to increase in cold damp weather and decrease in warm dry weather. This has given rise to the popular belief that rheumatism is more frequent in moist climates (such as in Britain) and almost non-existent in the Sahara Desert. This is, in fact, a myth; rheumatism is not less common in hot countries, but it does hurt less. Any well-defined type of rheumatism or arthritis – such as rheumatoid arthritis – is equally common in wet Britain and in the dry parts of North America. The reason that some Africans or any member of the less affluent nations suffer less from arthritis than inhabitants of the affluent countries is due purely to the shorter life expectancy of the former – they just don't live long enough to get serious rheumatic conditions! However, the myth is understandable for although emigration to a warmer country will not change the fundamental cause of the rheumatism, it *will* make the condition seem less painful which, after all, is what the sufferer is concerned about.

But emigration to Spain has a few snags and the vast costs of medical treatment will probably be only a minor consideration in comparison to the feasibility of such a therapeutic move. There are simpler methods of dealing with sensitivity to cold – which is often particularly intense for sufferers from low back pain – such as placing a hot water bottle on the back. Any cold draught or chilling may increase the pain and for some sufferers it may be impossible to get to sleep without a hot water bottle on the back, even in the summer.

Similar cold-sensitive pain occurs around the knee, particularly in women where one sometimes finds pads of discoloured fat which are cold to touch and tender. They may be one or two degrees in temperature cooler than the surrounding area when tested with a special thermometer.

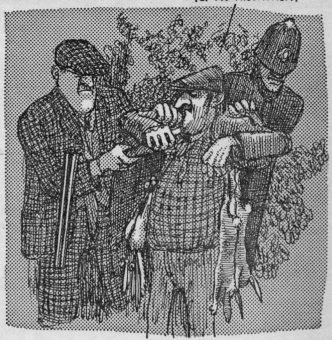

Cold-sensitive rheumatism is best treated with a close-fitting warm garment, as countless generations of hard-working peasants who do back-breaking work have found out. In Poland they wear rabbit skins on the back; in Southern France, Spain and Italy, wide woollen cummerbunds are part of the national peasant dress. In England, Doll's flannel is the traditional thing for a working man's backache, and modern equivalents include insulating thermal underwear such as angora wool vests.

Rheumatism due to poor blood supply

Intermittent claudication may develop in older people who have a poor blood supply to the legs due to a blockage of the arteries. It is present particularly in the calf muscles and comes on during walking and disappears with rest. A sufferer finds that when he goes for a walk he has to stop after about 100 yards or so and wait before he can proceed. It is due to the muscles using up the blood at a faster rate than it is being supplied because the arteries are silted up or narrowed. Many patients are cured without treatment as new arteries can grow, but usually the process takes several years. Expert vascular surgeons can sometimes help by providing a new 'spare part' artery.

Migraine is sometimes included amongst these rheumatic conditions. It is thought to be due to a spasm of an artery inside the head but, luckily, it is usually temporary.

Cramp is also probably due to poor blood supply. It rarely affects children unless their legs get cold and the blood vessels contract, as when swimming in cold water. But elderly people suffer from cramp, especially in bed at night. It is thought to be due to a build-up of local waste products in the muscle because the circulation does not get rid of them quickly enough. Consequently the muscle is stimulated to contract in a spasm and produce pain.

The traditional treatment for cramp is to take a tablet or two of quinine (the same drug as is used for malaria) before going to bed at night. This works very well for some older people and the cramp returns if they forget to take the tablets. But it does not seem to work so successfully for everybody. Another simple and often successful remedy is to take increased amounts of salt in the diet – this can be done by adding extra salt to all food and by drinking some salty soup last thing at night. But a warning is necessary for the elderly and people with a heart condition – they should not take extra salt except under a doctor's supervision, as it might be dangerous. A preferable alternative, which is equally effective, can be calcium salts.

The *Stitch* is thought to be due to cramp in part of the diaphragm of muscle which separates the abdomen from the thorax.

Proctalgia fugax is another painful cramp. This is a very severe pain which comes on with lightning-like rapidity and is felt in the back passage. Luckily, it only lasts for a second or so, but it still causes anxiety in some people who fear that they are developing a cancer. In fact, it is quite harmless.

Loose joints: an asset or liability?

Just as people vary in height, weight, hair, complexion and so on, so do they also vary in the suppleness and stiffness of their joints. There is just as much variation of agility in people as between racehorses and carthorses, greyhounds and bulldogs. Typically, Indians and Arabs tend to have suppler joints than Western Europeans, but there is of course, a good deal of individual variation in each race. Children are more supple than adults, and adults are more supple than old people. But with constant training and practice a dancer or athlete can keep the joints more supple than his or her contemporaries, even to the age of sixty or more.

However, some kinds of suppleness seem to be harmful and

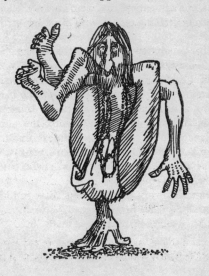

lead to injuries to joints and the soft tissues. Indeed in some, 'suppleness' is so severe that patients with it are defined as having diseases, running in the family. An example is 'Marfan's syndrome'; the affected person usually has very long fingers and toes and legs – quite disproportionately long in comparison to the height of the trunk. The muscles in this condition are relatively weak and the ligaments are so slack that the spine and joints can easily become deformed, dislocated or damaged.

But lesser degrees of hyperlaxity exist and may be partly an asset as well as partly a liability. Thus, in a study of American footballers, for example, it was discovered that an above average number of footballers had an unusual laxity of joints. In other words, lax-jointedness was associated with becoming a good athlete. At the same time, however, when the football injuries were counted up, it was found that the lax-jointed footballers had *more* than their share of injuries when compared to their normal fellow footballers. So, here again, lax-jointedness indicates a predisposition to injuries such as sprains. A similar study of English ballet dancers came to much the same conclusion; dancers when compared to nurses tended to display a laxity in all of their joints, including those that were not specifically stretched by the dancing training process. This suggested that lax-jointedness is one of the things that makes a girl a good dancer rather than that dancing causes the joints to become lax.

However, most of the 'rheumatic' problems of lax-jointedness occur in later life, if at all. People with over-supple feet tend to develop fallen arches which become painful; in others the knees which may to some extent bend back to front develop premature osteoarthrosis (Chapter 6); in the hands the supple-jointed person may, when young, be able to get his thumb to bend back so far that he can let it lie along the forearm, but because of this when he gets older the same thumb joint may become prematurely damaged and stiff.

The extreme forms of lax-jointedness are seen in some circus contortionists but these people usually also have exceptional muscle strength which helps to protect their joints.

9 Rheumatism in children

The legend referred to at the beginning of the first chapter states that it was the graceful antelope who decided to doom man the hunter – with the curse of rheumatism in his joints. But according to the legend, the antelope relented because of the beauty of man's children and modified the curse so that it should only affect man in adult life!

But children *do* get rheumatism. It is far less common than in adults and serious crippling rheumatism is almost unheard of, but nevertheless it does exist. The ratio of children who do suffer from a rheumatic attack of any kind is tiny in comparison to those that don't – if roughly one word in this chapter equals the child sufferer then all the other words represent the healthy children! But if you've had any experience of children you will know that the child who complains at one time or another of rheumatic pains is not nearly so rare. Mild temporary and unimportant aches and pains are so common that a special term – growing pains – has developed to embrace them all. One good way of distinguishing the serious from the unimportant types of rheumatism is by looking for swelling of the joints. If a child complains of an arm, a leg or a joint which is swollen, it is usually important. If the child complains of pain in the arm or leg but there is no swelling, it may be important but usually it is not.

This chapter will deal with:

1 mild, pretended and psychological rheumatism in children;

2 the two most well-known rheumatic conditions in children – Rheumatic Fever and Still's Disease;

3 the rarer causes of arthritis in children, including the attacks associated with certain diseases.

Foot problems in children are usually due to poorly fitting

shoes and often lead to painful feet in later life. They are dealt with in detail in the next chapter.

Aches and pains

Growing pains

Why do some children get growing pains? Quite often the explanation is simply that the child is seeking attention. 'Mummy, I can't get to sleep because my feet hurt' often means the same as 'I can't get to sleep; may I have a glass of water?' or 'Mummy, will you read me a story?' Mothers are naturally concerned about their children's health and many children soon learn that complaints about an arm or a leg hurting elicit more attention than other tried devices.

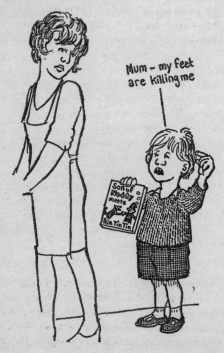

Sometimes the child is just copying the mother. The mother who says 'I must put my legs up, my feet are killing me' is associating the two ideas of lying down and having painful feet. Children are great mimics and they try out this idea. Their feet hurt too and they lie down. If this makes their mother concerned and sympathetic, they are more likely to do it again. And again and again. Until in desperation, the mother takes her child to a doctor.

If such complaints are recognized as just the equivalent of asking for a bedtime story, then the wise mother will read a bedtime story, not forgetting of course to look at the so-called painful limb to reassure the child and herself that there is nothing wrong. Handled this way, the child seldom complains for very long.

Handled some other way, the situation may build up until both mother and child are convinced of the onset of some terrible disease. The contrast of the doctor not being able to find

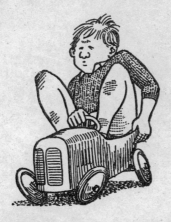

anything wrong may even increase the mother's worry. This type of situation is very common, particularly where there are sensitive and imaginative children and a mother who is prone to worrying. Girls seem more liable to become affected than boys, but it is usually nothing more than a phase in the child's development occurring between the ages of two and ten. Given tact and patience the 'growing pains' disappear in the same inexplicable way as they started. 'Growing pain' is not, strictly speaking, a medical term but many doctors use it because of the lack of any other name.

The fact that the joints are not swollen is a good indication that nothing serious is amiss. But occasionally the doctor may decide to prove that the complaints are nothing more than growing pains by asking for x-rays and blood tests. This helps to rule out any possibility of a serious disease since in growing pains there are no changes on the x-ray and the blood tests are normal. The danger here is in the effect this may have on the child. He or she, may be convinced that because a fuss is being made (x-rays and a prick in the arm) something *must* be wrong.

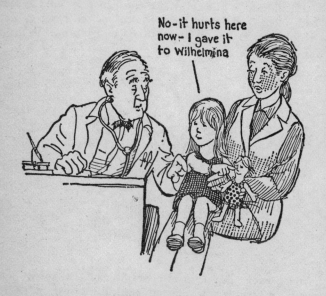

The wisest way for the doctor to handle this is to reassure the mother and child of his belief in the fact that nothing is wrong and explain that the tests are just routine.

Cold-sensitive pain

Another form of trivial rheumatism of which children often complain is pain in the feet and ankles during cold weather. This tends to affect boys more than girls; a typical situation is a boy of about ten or eleven years old standing around for a long time watching a football match in cold wet shoes. Even once he is home and is wearing dry shoes and socks, his feet may continue to ache for several hours. This isn't, of course, true rheumatism, it is merely cold-induced pain. For example, if you take a block of ice and hold it tightly in one hand for several minutes, your hand does not only feel cold, it also hurts. If you hold the ice longer, the pain becomes more and more severe and spreads up the arm until it is even felt in the chest. The pain, in this experiment, is due to the ice literally 'chilling the bones' inside the hand. Bones and other structures below the skin cannot feel cold, they can only feel pain.

People vary in their susceptibility to cold-induced pain. Some will notice little or no pain when they hold the ice cube. Similarly, in children, some feel pain whenever their legs are chilled whilst others hardly ever have this problem.

The answer, of course, is to avoid the situation which creates the aching – wear warm socks and waterproof shoes. However, if the feet do become chilled, a hot soak in a bath or a hot bottle in the bed will soon ease the aching.

Psychological or psychosomatic pains

Children occasionally complain of pain in their limbs as an expression of personal or family tension. This could arise from a feeling of insecurity such as some children have if their parents are continuously arguing. The doctor cannot do anything in this sort of situation; it is up to the parents to provide a peaceful home or temporarily send the child away. Or it could be because the child sleeps alone and has nightmares, or that he is bullied at school. Any number of events or circumstances could lead him to complain of pains rather than about the real cause of his worry. If the situation with regard to school bullying or nightmares is recognized, it may be possible to change it and stop the complaint.

These are some of the less important sorts of childhood rheumatism. The next section deals with the more serious kinds.

Rheumatic fever

The disappearance of rheumatic fever in this country has been one of the great medical victories of the last half-century. Around 1900 something like half of all the children admitted to the medical wards of the Hospital for Sick Children in Great Ormond Street were suffering from rheumatic fever and its complications. The Medical Research Council Rheumatism Unit at Taplow was originally set up in 1945 to deal with children suffering from this condition. Recently they have confidently been able to state that 'Rheumatic fever is now a rare and comparatively mild disease' and they are now concentrating their work on other forms of rheumatism in children. Unfortunately, this does not apply in less affluent countries such as Egypt, Mexico and India, where even today the wards are full of children suffering from severe rheumatism with heart disease.

The cause of rheumatic fever . . .
Rheumatic fever is one of the few rheumatic diseases for which the cause is known. It always follows an infection of the throat with a special kind of micro-organism, the haemolytic streptococcus, producing what is commonly known as a 'strep throat'. Having a 'strep throat' does not necessarily mean that the child will get rheumatic fever – even in the 'bad old days' no more than three per cent of strep throats were followed by rheumatic fever. Today thousands of children have strep throats without a single instance of rheumatic fever becoming apparent. But occasional patients with rheumatic fever do turn up and without exception they have evidence in their blood of having previously had streptococcal infection of the throat.

. . . and of its disappearance
Part of the disappearance of rheumatic fever may have been due to the availability of antibiotics such as penicillin. This has enabled prompt treatment of streptococcal infection of the

throat to which it is very sensitive. But this doesn't seem to be the whole answer and many scientists think that the general improvement in living standards has in some way increased our resistance. Others think that the organism itself has become less virulent.

What happens in rheumatic fever

Some seven to fourteen days after the throat infection the child who is going to get an attack becomes feverish and often looks pale and ill. One or more of the joints will swell and become painful. Often one joint swells when another one has just begun to improve, aptly named the 'flitting arthritis'. This arthritis and fever make it imperative to keep the child in bed. Other signs of an attack include the development of small nodules, which are about the size of a grain of wheat, on the elbows or knuckles and a peculiar rash on the arms and trunk.

Heart involvement

There is a saying that rheumatic fever 'licks the joints and bites the heart'. Certainly, the greatest threat in rheumatic fever is the possibility of involvement of the heart. This takes the form of an inflammation of the heart's three coats, the pericardium or outer coat, the myocardium or muscle, and the endocardium or lining.

Pericarditis. Inflammation of the outer coat of the heart may produce pain, usually felt in the front of the chest, spreading to the left shoulder. Breathing intensifies the pain and children sometimes become very short of breath with this.

Myocarditis. Direct inflammation of the muscle is seldom a serious cause of worry at this stage, but it does occur. One result is the development of an irregular pulse and other changes which can be picked up on the electrocardiogram. It is extremely rare for this to cause the heart actually to fail.

Endocarditis. Inflammation of the lining of the heart can involve the valves which may stretch and become inefficient. Years later, often after many attacks, the valves become thick and fail to open and close properly. This interferes with the heart's efficiency as a pump and if it is severe may lead to long-term disability from breathlessness.

St Vitus's Dance

One occasional accompaniment of rheumatic fever is chorea or St Vitus's Dance. This consists of involuntary movements and twitches, often starting in one side of the body. Because of this, the child appears clumsy and frequently drops things. And to make it worse, it is not unusual for children with this condition to find themselves being punished for breaking the crockery whilst washing up! Although it may persist for a long time it is not often serious and never leaves permanent changes.

Prevention

Most diseases of children, such as mumps, are the sort that leave an immunity so that once the child has had one attack, he becomes immune and will never develop another. But with rheumatic fever the situation is quite different. Once he has had one attack he is more liable to have another. To prevent recurrences a child may be given daily tablets of penicillin or a monthly injection of a long acting penicillin which will stop any fresh streptococcal sore throat.

If the heart has been involved in the child's first attack, then it is almost certain that there will be heart involvement in any recurrent attacks. But if he escaped it in the first attack he will escape it in further attacks. For this reason many doctors do not insist on long-term prevention of rheumatic fever in children who have never had any heart involvement. But they will usually insist that every new sore throat be promptly treated with penicillin or some other antibiotic to make sure that the organism doesn't get a fresh foothold.

The question of how long should prevention go on has no certain answer. Most authorities argue that children with rheumatic heart disease should continue taking penicillin for at least five years after the last attack or until leaving school or college – whichever is the longer.

Rheumatic heart disease

In those rare instances where a child has rheumatic fever and is left with rheumatic heart disease, the question arises 'Can anything be done?' Apart from preventing recurrences of rheumatic fever (which might make the heart trouble worse), it is also possible today by the use of surgery to correct some of the damage.

The commonest valve lesion 'mitral stenosis' – a narrowing of the mitral valve – is fairly easily corrected surgically. The next most frequent, 'mitral incompetence' is a widening of the valve base so that blood refluxes at each stroke of the heart beat. It can also be treated but is a little more difficult. The operation involves replacing the natural valve with an artificial one. Even more difficult, but now possible, is the ability to correct damage to the aortic valve. In some patients surgeons have successfully corrected both the mitral and the aortic valves in one operation.

One problem which should be mentioned here is that when teeth are extracted or filled, many of the bacterial organisms which normally live in the mouth are liberated into the blood stream for a short period. This infection is likely to settle in the heart valves damaged by rheumatic fever and could therefore be serious. For this reason, anyone with rheumatic heart disease should receive penicillin at the time of any dental treatment.

The tonsils and rheumatic fever

There is no evidence that removing the tonsils will make any difference to the rheumatism caused by 'strep throats'. But in fact, many sufferers need to have their tonsils removed purely because of the permanent damage and scarring that the numerous 'strep throats' have caused.

Juvenile chronic polyarthritis (Still's disease)

George Frederick Still was the first man to understand that there is a chronic form of arthritis in children which is not just a long-lasting variety of rheumatic fever. He was a physician at the Hospital for Sick Children in Great Ormond Street and in his time this particular disease – subsequently called after him – was

174 Rheumatism in children

much less common than rheumatic fever. It is still rare though it now probably seems more frequent because rheumatic fever has become so scarce.

Juvenile chronic polyarthritis, usually abbreviated to JCP, only occurs in about six in every ten thousand school children and in many of these cases it is only mild and passing. Eighty per cent recover completely, being left with minor changes which can only be detected by experts or by the use of x-rays; of those that go on to develop trouble in adult life, some manifest a condition which is indistinguishable from rheumatoid arthritis and some boys develop trouble in adult life which looks more like ankylosing spondylitis (see Chapter 2).

Three kinds of juvenile chronic polyarthritis

1 In one kind there is a swelling in one or two of the main joints. The knees and wrists in particular are affected. After a period of time – often long – the swelling clears up. The knee usually recovers completely but the wrist tends to stiffen up as it heals so that it won't move through its normal range.

2 Another common kind is similar to adult rheumatoid arthritis. The hands and feet are affected: the small joints of the fingers, toes, wrists and ankles swell up and, to some extent, the other larger joints may be troublesome as well. In the most severe cases of this variety, the neck, shoulders and hips are involved, which means that the children may become severely crippled.

3 The third main type starts as a persistent fever and illness in which there is often initially no joint trouble at all. It is only after some time that the joint disease develops and even then it is mild and it is the fever and general illness which dominate the picture.

These three kinds of JCP are not always so well defined in practice. There are also all sorts of intermediate varieties. But although it is possible that one kind will 'develop' into another usually it does not.

It is important to stress that JCP is not just rheumatism of the joints. Many other parts of the body can be affected.

The skin may show a peculiar sort of rash in the shape of little red blotches present in the mornings over the trunk and limbs and disappearing in the afternoons. The doctor who always does his visits after lunch may miss it. Other children develop swelling of the lymph glands in the neck and in the armpit. Some become anaemic. A few develop inflammation around the outer coat of the heart – pericarditis – similar to that which may occur in rheumatic fever, but not involving the lining and the valves of the heart.

Perhaps the most alarming complication is when the eyes become involved; inflammation of the iris may occasionally lead to blindness. This is very significant as this disease is one of the very few conditions which cause blindness in children.

A further, but very rare complication, is 'amyloidosis'. Amyloid is an inert material which gets deposited in the liver, spleen and kidneys and interferes with their functions.

Who is affected and why?

Nobody really knows what causes chronic polyarthritis in children. There is some evidence to imply that a tendency to get this condition is inherited. Boys with it tend to have more relatives with ankylosing spondylitis than chance would suggest. And, this in turn, is linked to the inherited white cell group, HLA B27 which we saw in Chapter 2 was present in almost all patients with ankylosing spondylitis. In twin studies, when one twin is affected, both members of identical twin pairs are more frequently affected than with non identical twin pairs, but it is obvious that inheritance does not provide us with a complete explanation. The truth is that we just do not know what the cause or causes are, particularly as it does not seem to be one single condition but several slightly different ones.

JCP can start early in life; the youngest recorded case is a baby of nine months. Girls are more frequently affected than boys, the ratio being about 2 : 1. Another feature is the broad variety of the victims; it is no respecter of the rich or the poor, both seem equally vulnerable. Nothing in the way of food that is eaten, exposure to damp, exercise or other illness seems particularly liable to bring it on.

Stunted growth

The fact that children are still growing when they contract what is otherwise an adult disease, radically affects the situation. Whatever the illness, a sick child usually fails to grow properly and a chronically sick child may end up shorter than his normal brothers and sisters. Also, the age of puberty will arrive later for the sick child.

The situation with JCP is even more worrying: when a joint is badly inflamed the growing part of the bone – which is near the joint – may be affected. At first, it may be stimulated so that the bone grows faster than normal. But subsequently it is often damaged so that it fails to grow. This can produce odd-looking results with one arm or leg shorter than the other, or one toe shorter than the rest.

In the past the problem was increased because cortisone and its derivatives, prednisone and many other similar drugs (see Chapter 4), which are often given for the relief of pain and inflammation, specifically act to stop growth, so that a child aged eight may be no taller than at age four when he or she first started taking tablets. The dilemma for the doctor was, should the child be given other weaker tablets which might not give such good pain relief but which would allow the child to grow more or less normally? Happily, this question is resolved today as it is now possible to use these drugs to provide good relief of pain and inflammation without the penalty of stunting, in all but the most severely affected children.

Treatment of Still's disease

Drugs: Drug treatment is similar to that given for adult rheumatoid arthritis. There are two classes of treatment.

1 There are the quick-acting tablets which relieve pain and inflammation. The simplest of these is aspirin, and the most powerful is cortisone and its derivatives.

2 The second class of tablets is concerned with long-term suppression of the illness. Gold injections and immuno-suppressive drugs are amongst those which can be given.

Children with severe disease usually need a drug of each class.

However, and this point needs to be stressed, the treatment does not just come out of a bottle. Many other things are vitally important:

Rest and exercise: It is important that children with Still's Disease have exactly the right amount of rest. It needs to be prescribed just like medicine – too much is as bad for them as too little. Joints which have become bent up may need plaster splints or an operation to get them straight. Complications like anaemia and amyloidosis may need to be tackled so as to improve the child's general resistance to disease. The most important kind of physiotherapy is probably the hot pool, where a hydrotherapist may teach the child to move the limbs again. Usually they do not need teaching – the children are delighted to have the chance of moving joints in warm water which, if moved on dry land, might be painful. In general, children need much less rest than adults and are much better when kept active, even if they have a temperature and their joints are swollen. But it is a matter for the expert to decide how much rest and exercise and how much splinting is necessary for each individual child.

Hospitalization and education: Child psychologists argue that whenever possible, a sick child should be admitted to a hospital near his home so that the parents can frequently visit him. But for some cases this is not the only consideration. A crippled child will have to learn to work with his head rather than with his hands and so it is vitally important that he gets his schooling and passes his exams. Whenever possible doctors will arrange treatment and headmasters will cooperate in order to try and keep the child in his normal school, even if he cannot keep up with all his class mates. But for the more severely disabled child who has to go into hospital for a longer period, hospital schools are available particularly in those centres which specialize in rheumatism in children.

With the advances in understanding about the various kinds of chronic arthritis in childhood, it has become important to obtain the correct diagnosis and treatment. Special centres have been or are being set up in Taplow, Manchester and Bath.

Surgery: It is occasionally necessary to operate on damaged joints. The most common operations are on the hips, knees and wrists to prevent stiffening or correct deformities. Artificial hips have now been successfully put into adolescents and a great deal can be done by surgeons to correct bad positions of the knees and wrists. But such operations are rarely needed these days. Children are in many ways much tougher than adults. They have a remarkable ability to recover from what often seem impossible circumstances, including being affected by a devastating disease.

The future: Very few children with juvenile chronic polyarthritis actually die of it. Most grow up and lead normal lives. They may end up being rather shorter than their school fellows but their intelligence is not affected. They get married and have children. Since there is no strong evidence that the condition is directly inherited, there is no need for them to worry about passing it on to their children.

Rarer causes of arthritis in children

There are a large number of rarer causes of arthritis and joint disease in children and only a few of them will be considered here. It is often difficult to distinguish one from another and a skilled specialist has to be called in to give the diagnosis.

The same problem sometimes exists in sorting out rheumatic illnesses from some of the commoner childhood diseases. Any child who is developing a feverish illness is liable to get aches and pains in the back and limbs, especially when the temperature is going up. The child will usually look ill, may vomit, shiver and have a hot forehead even if the hands and feet look pale and feel cold. This sort of rheumatism is particularly common before the onset of measles and German Measles. But it may precede any of the childhood fevers such as mumps and chickenpox. The pains often arrive several days before the rash appears (in measles or chickenpox) or before the glands swell (in mumps). Except in an epidemic, even the doctor may find it difficult to say what illness the child is developing in this early stage of fever and aches and pains in the limbs.

Meningitis

A word of warning is needed. If the aches and pains are accompanied by pains in the back and neck, and particularly if the neck is so stiff that the child cannot bring his head forwards on to his chest, it may be due to an infection of the brain. In meningitis (cerebro-spinal fever) and in poliomyelitis (infantile paralysis) headache and stiff neck are common early in the illness. In poliomyelitis this is often accompanied by quite severe pains in one or other of the limbs.

Henoch Schonlein Purpura

Henoch Schonlein Purpura is the rather magnificent name for a rare cause of arthritis which accompanies a characteristic rash. The child becomes feverish then develops the rash which is particularly obvious on areas that are subjected to pressure; if the child is lying in bed, then the buttocks are likely to be affected. The peculiarity of this rash is that in the middle of the red spots there are purple blotches caused by bleeding under the skin. Such children frequently suffer from attacks – often quite severe – of pain in the abdomen. This is thought to be due to bleeding in or around the gut. Another feature of this condition is that the children develop an arthritis similar to rheumatic fever, but they do not get heart problems. The arthritis is usually mild, transient and of no serious importance. The disease is only serious if it continues for a long time and only then if it involves the kidneys – causing a high blood pressure – or the eyes – causing bleeding inside the eyeball, which may lead to blindness.

Treatment is in the form of cortisone or its derivates, but it is only needed for severe cases. If the eyes or kidneys become diseased, the immunosuppressive drugs (see Chapter 4) may then be prescribed.

German measles

In some epidemics of German measles (rubella) those affected develop a true arthritis and not just the aches and pains of a fever. Some of the larger joints in the body swell up and become painful. This may last for several weeks or even a month or two, but it practically always seems to clear up. It is therefore a relatively trivial problem.

Erythema nodosum

Another childhood skin condition which is sometimes associated with a type of arthritis is erythema nodosum. This strange sounding name refers to a painful blotchy rash which appears on the shins in the form of reddish lumpy swellings. These are tender to touch and eventually show deep bruising. In itself this is a trivial condition and the arthritis which accompanies it is usually transient, but the doctor will want to investigate it thoroughly as it is occasionally caused by some other more serious internal disease.

Psoriasis

Chapter 5 described in some detail the different ways in which psoriasis can be associated with arthritis in adults. The first attack of psoriasis – which appears as a persistent rash consisting of angry red patches covered with silvery scales – often occurs in childhood. When it does, there is about a five per cent chance that it will be accompanied by a form of arthritis similar to juvenile chronic polyarthritis. The problems and treatment are much the same.

Haemophilia

It is common knowledge that haemophilia is a bleeding disease, but the fact that it is also a disease of the joints is not so widely known. It is one of the few conditions that is definitely inherited, and as such it has a 'royal history'.

Descendants of Queen Victoria married into the Russian and Spanish royal families and transmitted the disease there. Crown Prince Alexei, heir to the Czar of Russia during the First World War, was subject to disastrous episodes of bleeding into his joints. Because of this, as many old pictures show, he was carried around on the shoulders of a sailor in the Czar's Navy. The monk Rasputin claimed to be able to stop the bleeding and because of this exercised an extraordinary influence over the boy's mother, the Czarina, Alexandra. All perished in the Russian revolution.

Haemophilia only affects boys, but women can transmit the disease to their sons. A daughter of a haemophiliac has a fifty per cent chance of becoming a carrier.

Characteristically, boys who are affected will bleed for a long time even after mild wounds. Some boy babies have died from continuous bleeding after circumcision. Other patients have difficulty in stopping bleeding after a tooth has been extracted. But while mild cases just show prolonged bleeding, the more severely affected bleed under the skin into the muscles or joints. This can cause deformity and crippling.

Preventing joint damage is now possible for patients with haemophilia. Although it cannot be cured, it can be treated. If normal blood is separated into plasma and red cells and the plasma is put in a cold refrigerator under certain conditions, some solid material settles out of it and is known as 'cryoprecipitate'. It contains the particular substances which are deficient in haemophiliac boys. If cryoprecipitate is given promptly to the boy, it will stop the bleeding immediately.

Blood collected in Blood Transfusion Centres is much too precious to use directly. It, or most of it, is separated into the red cells and plasma. The plasma in turn is separated into all the many different factors which are useful to Medicine. One of these is Factor VIII – the anti-haemophilia factor. Today haemophiliacs are often given injections of purified Factor VIII.

It is therefore most important for the family with a haemophiliac child to live near one of the major haemophilia centres. The parents of such children are often given the privilege of calling the ambulance themselves to take the child direct to the Centre if bleeding is suspected, without first trying to get hold of the family doctor. The more practical and intelligent parents can be taught to give an intravenous injection of Factor VIII. This can be kept for emergencies in the family refrigerator. A useful temporary measure which can also be kept in the refrigerator is the instant cold pack, a plastic bag full of a material which will not freeze. When this is placed over a joint that has been the subject of bleeding it can relieve pain and will probably stop the bleeding until other help arrives.

Today the greatest enemy of the haemophiliac is the car accident. Ironically, once joint damage has occurred, the sufferers are even more dependent than the rest of us on car transport, but even a minor accident may be dangerous for a haemophiliac. The statistics are daunting for us all – the probability of one car accident for every 80,000 miles driven by the average motorist in Britain – but for the haemophiliac they are frightening and alarming. As a precaution all haemophiliacs should carry a special identity card which gives their disease and blood group in case they need an emergency transfusion.

Vitamin deficiencies

Scurvy develops in babies when there is a deficiency in the diet of Vitamin C. This may occur if the child has been kept on artificial milk feeds for too long without being given orange juice or any other source of Vitamin C. As a result, there is a tendency for bleeding in and around the joints. This is very painful, but luckily the condition is usually quite apparent to a skilled paediatrician.

Rickets is another vitamin deficiency disease which causes trouble to joints. In this case it is due to a deficiency of Vitamin D, the sunshine vitamin. Such children tend to be stunted, their arms and legs grow 'bent' and their joints may feel painful. Curing rickets is usually straightforward but a few children may need enormous doses of Vitamin D as they are resistant to it. However, too much Vitamin D can also be bad and blood tests are needed to check that the right dose is being used.

Bone diseases

Many bone diseases in children initially appear to be a form of rheumatism. The most serious is an infection of the bone – osteomyelitis. If the infection is located near to the joint the child will often complain of pain in the joint. It is usually very painful and causes the child to become generally ill and have a fever. Diagnosis can be difficult as X-rays do not show any changes until late in the disease. It may be necessary to prescribe antibiotic treatment without having tracked down which organism is responsible.

Leukaemia

Leukaemia in children sometimes presents itself as a form of 'rheumatism'. This is because the bone marrow near to the joints may become involved and thus irritate the joints. The joint may swell and, of course, the bones nearby will become painful. Important medical advances have been made, making it possible to prolong the lives of children who are affected by leukaemia and in relieving much of their suffering.

Preventing arthritis and rheumatism in adult life

Some children are born with *congenital dislocation of the hip*. The hip is not correctly positioned in its socket. If they are allowed to walk like this, they will develop lifelong deformities and a peculiar waddling gait. Today paediatricians examine newborn babies for dislocation of the hip; if this is detected the position of the hip can be corrected and the child nursed in a special splint until the hip stays in its socket in a normal manner.

Another condition which, if treated when the patient is young, will prevent permanent damage is *Perthe's Disease*. This is a disease of adolescent children in which the growing part of the bone near the hip joint becomes damaged. It usually occurs in rather overweight children. They complain of pain in the groin and begin to limp. If treated early, the condition may settle down without any serious after-effects; but if neglected the hip joint may be permanently damaged so that serious trouble arises in later life.

10 Painful feet

The structure of the human foot, bone for bone and joint for joint, is very similar to the human hand. But there the resemblance ends. We cannot possibly do the same things with the feet as with the hands, or vice versa. For example, we cannot grasp objects or play the piano with our toes, neither can the hands bear the weight of the body for more than a few minutes. We marvel at the weightlifter who is able to use his hands to lift several times his own body weight above his head for a few seconds. We forget that the same man's feet have to carry the same amount of weight plus the weight of his body. Moreover the feet – which are constructed in the same way as the hand – must carry the body weight all day and every day.

The hand is on show; gloves are worn only for protection against hard work or weather. The foot is usually hidden; coverings of socks, stockings and shoes prevent exposure. The hand is free to move in any direction; the foot is cramped in its containers. Rings are worn to accentuate the delicate appearance of the female hand; the foot is often considered to be unattractive, dirty and smelly. Consequently, more concern is given to the shoe. Far too many people, particularly young women, buy shoes primarily to be 'in fashion' and do not worry about whether they actually fit. It is inevitable that such people will be affected later on by a number of unnecessary and often uncomfortable troubles in their feet. These may have nothing to do with rheumatism, but if rheumatism or arthritis does develop in the feet, it is not just a question of discomfort but of serious, painful and crippling deformity. The possibility should never be dismissed as unlikely. After all, there are over twenty joints in each foot and any one, or all of them, can be affected by arthritis.

The anatomy of the foot

The structure

One of the most important but least considered parts of the foot is the curious fibrous and fatty cushion which separates the sole from the bones. It is the structure of this which enables the foot to bear enormous pressures.

The soles of people who don't wear shoes become horny and thick until the skin is just like tough leather. In fact, to be accurate, it *is* tough leather! People who wear shoes have thinner soles but the skin is still very tough. Between this skin and the bony skeleton inside there is a sponge-like feltwork of fibres. The spaces between the fibres are filled in with soft fat which forms the cushions of the heel and under the joints at the base of the toes.

The bones of the feet are arranged in two so-called arches, the longitudinal and the transverse arch. The 'longitudinal

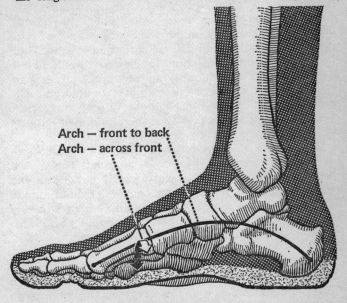

Arch — front to back
Arch — across front

The two arches of the foot

arch' describes the bones from the heel to the base of the toes. This supports the bones of the lower leg. The height of the arch varies enormously. It is possible to have either a high arch or a flat one which only appears whilst the person is standing on tiptoe – both are normal. It is also quite normal for toddlers to have very flat feet. The 'transverse' arch refers to the bones at the front of the foot. The five bones at the base of the toes are arranged so that it is mainly the big toe joint which takes the weight, supported to some extent by the bones of the little toe joint. In between, the bones form an arch which is able to support weight in abnormal conditions, or when the foot is under strain as in jumping or running, but they do not normally do so.

The muscles, tendons and ligaments are situated around the bones and allow for the 'springiness' and suppleness of the foot.

The development

A baby's foot is full of fat and without much structure. The foot of a growing child is very supple and mobile. Its potential to develop in the same way as the hand is indicated in the feet of those unfortunate children who are born without arms. Their feet develop almost as a substitute for the lack of hands, so that they can do with their toes what can only normally be done by the fingers. This supple and trainable foot of the child, gradually turns into the stiffer foot of adult life which is unable to function in any way other than that for which it is always used – namely taking the weight of the body.

Even in adult life, however, people's feet differ in the degree of stiffness or suppleness of the inside structures. This is often very significant. Two people may have exactly the same size and shape of foot at rest; but one person can have a rigid foot and so need a shoe that is an exact fit, whereas the other person may have a supple foot and can probably wear a shoe which is too small or the wrong shape, and feel little or no pain.

The nerve supply

The feet are second only to the hands in the richness of the nerve supply from the brain. This means that they are sensitive structures which if damaged are capable of giving rise to a great deal of pain. Even touching the skin can cause an unpleasant sensation – there are tales of a Chinese torture which consists of tickling the feet for several hours at a time! As in other parts of the body, the hard parts of the joints do not contain any pain nerve endings but the ligaments, tendons and skin around the joints are rich in pain fibres. This is particularly true of the skin around the nails.

The nerves to the feet also control the extent of sweating of the foot. Again, the wide variation between people's 'sweating feet' is quite normal. In a moist, sweaty foot the skin macerates and decomposes. The process is in fact similar to the rotting of moist leaves in a compost heap and is brought about by germs. The structure of the skin changes and becomes softer – it can often be scraped off between the toes and around the nails. At the same time the decomposition produces the characteristic 'cheesy' foot odours. Although the smell is an old problem, in modern days it is probably more severe! The reason for this is that such odours are more common in feet shod with impermeable shoes made of modern plastics than in feet shod in traditional leather which to some extent allows the foot to 'breathe'.

The blood supply

The foot has a good blood supply carried by two main arteries, one coming down in front of the ankle and one behind the ankle bone on the inner side of the heel. In older people and in diabetics, this circulation often fails. It is possible for it to block up completely, in which case there is considerable pain and there may even be gangrene due to loss of the blood supply. Diabetes with loss of blood supply is one of the main causes of leg amputation. Most of these patients, and it amounts to between three and four thousand in any one year, will have suffered severe foot pain before the decision is finally made to amputate and to seek the help of one of the artificial limb centres in this country. This pain is often initially attributed to 'rheumatism'.

Shoes and foot deformity

Barefoot in the park!

Shoes cause more foot problems than anything else and faulty shoes are especially to blame. If we didn't wear shoes there would probably be about ninety per cent less of the foot troubles that are suffered from today. But if we did go around barefoot there would no doubt be pain from other sources: frost bite in cold climates; cuts from thorns and sharp stones; bites from insects and snakes; infestation in tropical countries from certain sorts of parasitic worms. Ideally, the child should grow up in an always equable climate and do nothing but run around in bare feet on a grass lawn all day! He would presumably grow up without any foot deformities at all. But this idyllic situation just does not exist. We have to wear shoes to protect our feet and to that extent we have to accept that a certain number of foot deformities are likely to be with us however much we attempt to avoid them.

Aching feet – a common problem?

May Clarke, in her survey of the feet of a sample of British people in 1969, estimated that at least fifty per cent, and possibly eighty per cent, of the people of this country had something the matter with their feet. Most of these disorders were relatively trivial, such as ingrowing toenails, corns, athlete's foot or minor bunion joints. But there were also serious problems, particularly in older women. For them, foot deformities and nail problems constitute a major source of pain and disability. There are probably no more than two or three in every hundred women who have reached the age of eighty and still have 'normal' feet. Arthritis of the feet is far less common but the intense problems that it causes are much greater. From various estimates it is possible to guess that about two per cent of the adult population, which means nearly a million people, suffer from arthritis of the feet. At least nine out of every ten rheumatoid arthritics have trouble with their feet, whereas the hands are affected in only seven out of every ten.

Foot development – from dainty to deformed

How do the perfect pretty little feet of the baby become the rather unpleasant objects which support the weight of the adult? At what stage do deformities start and how can they be prevented? And once a deformity has developed, is it possible to re-straighten the foot?

The infant's foot until about the age of ten is a rapidly growing structure that is very soft and mobile. It is a mistake to view the baby's foot as a miniature adult foot, for it has a different shape. This means that the shape of a baby's shoe must not imitate the shape of an adult's shoe. It is particularly important for the child's shoe to have a straight inner border and be long

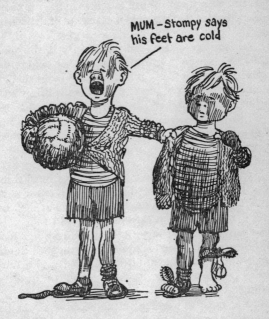

MUM – Stompy says his feet are cold

enough to allow the toes to wriggle inside the toe cap. As the toddler grows he may still crawl as much as he walks and his shoes will wear out as quickly on top as on the sole. From the age of four upwards, boys are particularly heavy on their shoes; few small boys can resist playing football in their best shoes. This is, in fact, a blessing in disguise, since it means that the shoes wear quickly and have to be replaced. Girls are often less fortunate; because they take longer to wear their shoes out, they tend to continue wearing the same shoes for longer periods. This means that the foot often outgrows the shoe and is one of the reasons why girls get more foot deformities than boys.

The first foot deformities begin in infancy with the tucking-in of the little toe under the fourth toe. This is probably due to tight socks and shoes which even if they don't seem too tight, nevertheless compress the toes. However, foot deformities at this age, and even up to the age of ten or more, are completely reversible provided that the child is taken out of the constriction of socks and shoes.

But after the age of ten, and particularly in the adolescent ages for girls between twelve and sixteen, shoe deformities tend to become permanent. Also, it is in this age range that girls are first prone to develop the sort of deformities which plague them throughout their adult lives. It is a critical time; their feet may grow by as much as half an inch in six months, but because children's feet are relatively insensitive they may wear tight shoes without complaint.

New shoes are expensive but so are old ones – in a different way. If the toes are cramped together during the vital finishing stage of the development of the foot, they are then moulded crooked for life. It is at this stage that the bunion joint forms, or the small toes become packed together and sooner or later become painful. The survey of schoolchildren's feet conducted by Dr Catherine Hollman found that over half of all children had a bunion joint by the age of fifteen and that girls were affected three times as often as boys.

In order to prevent this, barefoot activities should be encouraged as often as possible on the beach or in the fields, or even in the streets, and especially in the home. Whenever there is no danger to feet from cold weather, thorns or stones, children should be encouraged to do without shoes and in the summer to wear open-toed sandals. Tight socks are a special hazard. A wool sock that has shrunk, the nylon stretch sock or just simply a cotton sock that has been outgrown – any of these can bend the little toe against the others and sometimes right under or over the fourth toe. It is particularly important not to try and make shoes last too long at the stage when the child's foot is growing rapidly. For this reason, cheap shoes are often better than expensive ones since the temptation to make them last is not so great.

The worst offender for deforming girls' feet is the type of court shoe in which the shoes only stay on the foot because of the grip on the toes – this necessarily packs the toes together. Young girls, already fashion-conscious but unfortunately not health-conscious, only too readily try to force their feet into shoes which they regard as elegant. As a result, their feet become inelegant!

Deformities in the growing foot

There is a long list of deformities caused by badly fitting shoes worn on the growing foot. First the nails suffer. *Ingrowing toenails* are caused by pressure across the big toe and are often accompanied by deformities of other toenails. The joints of the big toe suffer with the development of a *bunion* which doctors call *hallux valgus*. The other toes develop a *hammer toe* deformity. The fifth toe is often pushed across to form a *bunionette*. The abnormal shape of the foot may mean that pressures develop between the skin and the shoe causing *corns*. Other pressures on the foot may cause an exaggeration or loss of the springy arches of the foot, again with the later development of pain.

The ideal shoe

Shoes which are suitable for children will not compress the toes and will leave room for toe action. They will have a straight inner border so that the big toe can lie in line with the inner side of the foot. They will clasp the heel reasonably firmly from side to side, and they will have something across the top, usually lacing, which will prevent the foot from sliding forwards in the

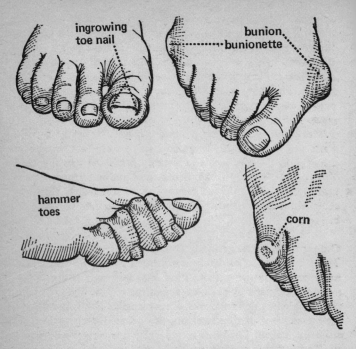

Common toe problems

shoe during walking or running. They will have a heel which is large enough to spread the weight of the body over a wide area.

Pain in the front part of the foot

Metatarsalgia: Middle-aged and elderly people may feel pain in the front part of the foot when they walk. This is called 'metatarsalgia' and is a direct result of a flattening of the anterior arch of the foot so that painful callosities form beneath the head of the second and third metatarsal bones. It is seldom the only foot deformity. Most sufferers have, or previously have had, hallux valgus or bunion joints. This sometimes means that people

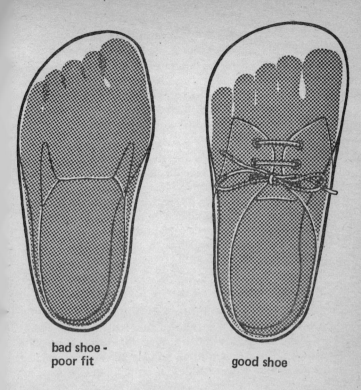

bad shoe -
poor fit

good shoe

weather the rather painful operations to have their hallux valgus removed, and are then disappointed to find that their feet are still in pain. This is because most operations for hallux valgus help to destroy the anterior arch of the foot and so more weight is placed on the other bones. And if the vital fibro-fatty cushion is not very thick under these other bones, then pain will result.

Morton's metatarsalgia: A special kind of metatarsalgia is called 'Morton's metatarsalgia'. In this condition one of the nerves to the toes gets nipped when it passes down in the cleft between the bones at the base of the toes. This is usually between the second and third toes. It can, of course, be extremely painful and is often associated with numbness of the skin on the sides of the toes. An operation may be needed to relieve the pain.

March fracture: Another painful condition in the forefoot is 'March fracture'. This refers to a fracture in one of the metatarsal bones. It occurs for no obvious reason and can happen in healthy young men as well as in older patients who have some form of generalized weakness of their bones. The pain is acute and the condition is often misdiagnosed as arthritis, but an x-ray will immediately pinpoint the trouble.

Frieberg's disease: 'Frieberg's disease' is a curious degeneration of part of the bone at the base of the second toe in children's feet. The onset of this condition is thought to occur after there has been some local damage. Again, the diagnosis can easily be made by x-ray but the condition is not treatable except for protecting the foot until the discomfort disappears. Fortunately, most cases become painless although they may lead to some deformity of the joint.

Pain in the middle part of the foot

Flat feet: Flat feet are neither necessarily abnormal nor painful. The majority of flat feet in children are probably harmless and don't need treating. Very often such a child has a very mobile foot and the 'flat' appearance only occurs when they are standing – as soon as they begin to walk, run or jump, the flat foot dis-

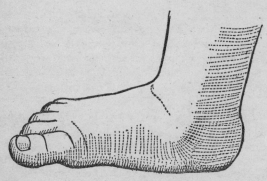

The normal 'flat' foot in children

appears. The appearance of a flat foot is sometimes due to a child having a short Achilles tendon at the back of the heel. The child (usually a girl) can only stand barefoot if she lets the ankles fall inwards. But few children have trouble in later life because their feet were flat as children. Indeed, several of them have ultimately become famous runners.

There is, however, one kind of flat foot in childhood which *is* painful and does need treatment. This is a fairly uncommon abnormality of growth in which two bones which should be separate in the foot are in fact joined by a bony bar. This produces pain from time to time and is called spastic flat foot.

High arched feet: The opposite of flat foot is an arch which is very high – called 'pes cavus' by doctors. A person with pes cavus leaves a footprint which consists only of an unjoined print of the heel and the front of the foot. Often such a foot is only one end of the continuum of a 'normal foot.' However, it is often associated with a hammer toe deformity and later with pressure lesions forming on the top of the clawed toes. There may also be problems from pressure beneath the toe joints since they are taking all the weight. Sometimes this high arch is so severe as to be a deformity of the foot and it may result from diseases of the nerves which have caused a weakness or a contracture of the muscles to the foot. Poliomyelitis is one such cause.

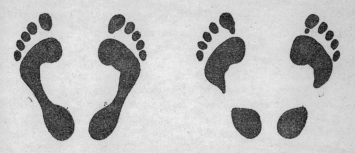

Prints from normal and high arched feet

Pain in the back of the foot

There are only two conditions which commonly arise in the back of the foot – plantar fasciitis and calcaneal bursitis.

Plantar fasciitis: 'Plantar fasciitis' means inflammation of the strong flat ligament, the 'plantar fascia', that runs from the heel bone to the toe bones along the sole of the foot. If you can imagine the foot as a bow, then this ligament acts like the string keeping it tight and maintaining the arch. The place where the fascia joins the bone at the heel, that is the enthesis*, often becomes strained and therefore painful. This condition is seen more often in men than in women and is sometimes a part of the abnormalities which accompany various forms of arthritis.

The treatment of this can be quite difficult. Some patients respond quite well to putting a large ring-shaped pad made of thick felt inside the heel. The hole in the ring corresponds to the tender area. By using this, all the pressure is taken off the painful area and so can be sufficient to allow it to mend. Sometimes the tender spot can be injected with cortisone. On other occasions even x-ray treatment or surgery may be needed.

Calcaneal bursitis: The other part of the heel which quite frequently hurts is the area at the back where the strong Achilles tendon is attached. Again, this can develop as part of a generalized arthritis but it often occurs on its own. Suitable padding and injection treatment will usually relieve the pain to a reasonable extent. It is called 'calcaneal bursitis' since it seems primarily to affect the little bursa or cushion that prevents the Achilles tendon and the back of the heel from rubbing.

There are various other, not so common, causes of pain around the heel and ankle. For example, the strong tendons which transmit the forces of the muscles in the calf down to the foot and the toes, all have to take a sharp turning around the ankle and to do this they pass through smooth slippery tunnels known as synovial sheaths. These sheaths can become inflamed and distended with fluid, often as part of a generalized arthritis.

* See Chapter 8 for a description of the enthesis

The foot in old age

Old people are particularly liable to have trouble with their feet. The foot, just like other parts of the body, changes with age. The skin under the foot becomes thin and not so elastic. The ligaments inside the foot become stiff and the whole foot structure becomes relatively rigid. The nails, although they grow slowly, tend to thicken and become hard to cut. Shoe deformities, such as bunion joints, gradually tend to get worse with age until the foot as well as being stiffer is also a good deal wider. If a person had a wide foot when young, then it may become impossible to find ready-made shoes which will fit the even wider foot. Add to this the difficulties of poor eyesight and the difficulties involved in stooping down to cut toenails or clean the toes, and it is then easy to see why many old people have a major problem with their feet.

The foot in arthritis

It has already been mentioned earlier in this chapter that nine out of ten people with rheumatoid arthritis get involvement of the joints of the feet. The joints most frequently affected are those at the base of the toes. Initially, they swell up causing the whole of the front of the foot to be both wider and thicker. A patient with rheumatoid arthritis usually needs to wear shoes that are at least two sizes wider and often one size longer in order to allow enough room for the swollen foot. As a result, many women who develop rheumatoid arthritis have drawers and cupboards full of shoes which they have bought hoping for comfort and which they can no longer wear.

At the back of the foot, the joint most frequently affected in arthritis is the joint beneath the ankle that allows the heel to twist inwards and outwards. If no treatment is given for this, the ankles appear to drop inwards.

In later rheumatoid arthritis the structure of the joints at the base of the toes softens, causing characteristic deformities from the pressures of standing and of wearing shoes. Hallux valgus or a bunion joint may become very severe. The smaller toes can be

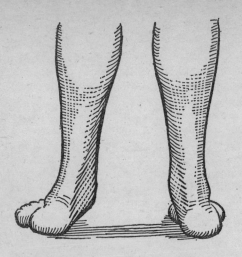

Bending in of the ankle and out of the heel

partially or completely dislocated at the joints at the base of the toe. Arthritis may also attack the bone near the joint so that it becomes rough or sharp and digs into the skin from inside.

More significant, however, is that the important fibro-fatty cushion moves forwards away from the weight-bearing area so that only relatively thin skin separates the damaged joints from the ground. This skin typically reacts by producing corns or callosities which are often painful. At the same time, other callosities form on the tops of the toe near the nails, where the weight is being carried right on the point of the bone. In addition, more callosities are forming on top of the 'knuckles' of the toes as they rub on the shoes. Because of the softening of the joints and the pressure of shoes, the smaller toes pack together in bizarre ways. Sometimes the little toe twists right underneath the others, sometimes it rides above them and the whole shape of the foot is distorted.

The later stages of arthritis in the back of the foot involve permanent deformity of the heel. Seen from the back of the foot

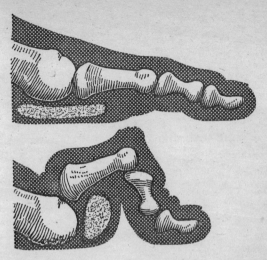

Dislocation of the toe joints and slipping forwards of the protective pad

it is quite clear how this upsets the way in which the weight of the body is carried down to the foot. Instead of the heel being in line with the leg, it is now displaced outwards and the ankle inwards. The weight of the body tends to aggravate the deformity. It may need a special brace with a sling, known as a T-strap, to prevent it becoming worse.

In the other forms of arthritis, those caused by ankylosing spondylitis, Reiter's syndrome, and the kind associated with psoriasis, the deformities of the foot are rather similar, although the pattern of involvement of the various parts of the foot tends to be a little different.

The foot in diabetes

If arthritis is the biggest cause of foot troubles, it is closely followed by diabetes. Diabetes is complicated by three factors, all of which may affect the feet.

1 The first is a tendency to a hardening and eventually to blocking of arteries. This may lead to loss of normal blood supply to the foot.

2 The second is a tendency to infection. Micro-organisms seem to thrive on the increased amount of sugar in the blood in diabetes.

3 The third is less well known but in many cases it is the most important. This is the tendency for the nerve supply to be interfered with so that the patient doesn't have the proper or appropriate sensations of pain. It is known as the 'diabetic neuropathic foot'.

Because of the diabetes, there is interference in the conduction of the smallest nerve fibres which carry pain messages and control the sweating and circulation. This usually only occurs in severe diabetics but occasionally can be the first sign of this condition. Because of this failure to feel pain, in a bad case a patient may not realize that he is continuing to walk with a nail sticking through the sole of the shoe. Or the toes may be rubbing in an ill-fitting shoe. Sooner or later the skin breaks down, infection gets in and a nasty ulcer, known as a penetrating ulcer, appears. If nothing is done and the patient continues to walk – as well he may because it doesn't hurt him – then the ulcer develops a spreading infection tunnelling right into the structure of the foot. It may eventually almost destroy the foot.

Another problem is the development of fractures. A patient not knowing that he has hurt himself may continue to walk, and a small crack in the bone will progress to form an actual fracture which still elicits little or no pain.

This is not to say that diabetic patients with this problem don't get any pain in their feet at all. An ulcer which has started in a painless part of the foot may cause a great deal of pain when infection spreads to another part of the foot which is still capable of sending pain messages.

It follows that diabetics who have this complication need to exercise great care. They are advised to have a mirror in the bathroom which is placed on the floor and to inspect the soles of the feet regularly for any sores or raw areas; they must feel inside their shoes every day before putting them on to make sure that no nail or small piece of stone has got in. Their shoes must be soft and wide enough to give plenty of room and if the shoe is to protect the foot, it must be kept dry. This means that diabetes is a special hazard for farmers and farmworkers. They commonly wear rubber boots to keep their feet dry, but rubber boots which they can get into may be quite the wrong shape for their feet and may rapidly cause ulcers on the feet and deformities of the joints.

Leprosy

The situation in diabetes is very similar to what happens to the feet in leprosy where infection of the nerves to the arms and legs causes loss of pain sensation. The deformities of the hands and feet in leprosy are directly due to this loss of the feeling of pain. Somebody afflicted by leprosy can hold a hot pan or a cigarette so that it burns him without even knowing. This, in turn, causes the flesh, and eventually the bones, to ulcerate and disappear. Leprosy can now be cured but in less affluent countries, with the rapid increase in population, the infection is spreading quicker than attempts to cure it can keep pace. Indeed, when one considers how leprosy can cause destruction of joints in fingers and feet, there is a good reason to make the startling statement that leprosy is probably now one of the most serious joint diseases in the world.

Treatment
The role of the chiropodist
Modern chiropodists are highly trained. As with other professions, there are specialists amongst them; some concentrate on the provision of beautifully moulded foot appliances, others

on providing special shoes, and others on the techniques of massage, manipulation and remedial exercises for the foot. But most of 'general practice chiropody' is concerned with the day-to-day care of the forefoot in older people – the cutting and cleaning of awkward toe-nails, the care and the dressings for corns and callosities, the provision of pads to help feet in pain from bunion joints or metatarsalgia. Most of these foot deformities are avoidable; they are the result of badly fitting shoes, weak foot muscles or too much pressure due to obesity. They create an unfortunate burden for chiropodists who are in short supply and are needed for other problems which are not yet preventable, such as the problems of arthritis in the feet or inherited deformities.

Arthritis in the feet: The main ways in which the chiropodist can help patients with arthritis of the feet are:

1 Ring pads. These take pressure off painful bony prominences by padding all round the area. The prominence goes through a hole in the middle. It is a common mistake for people trying to pad their own feet to put the padding on top of the prominence – this will only increase the pressure. The most suitable ring pads for bunion joints are made in the shape of a horseshoe out of thick adhesive felt. Smaller ring pads for the knuckles of the toes are usually bought ready-made. Alternatively, the toes may be bound in animal wool which not only protects them but, because it is slippery, allows the sock or shoe to move over the painful area.

2 Toe pads. These are put between or under the toes to 'prop' them into a better position. The painful callosities on the tips of clawed toes can often be corrected by a simple roll pad which the toes can grasp.

3 Metatarsal supports. Probably the most useful contribution of the chiropodist concerns the various kinds of metatarsal support. These are pads designed to take the weight of the body off the painful joints at the base of the toes and transfer it further back onto the soft parts of the foot. This is usually done by

strapping specially made pads on to the foot. The disadvantage of this method is that the pads have to be removed for washing and then replaced – this can often be a long and complicated job.

In some patients, however, these pads are placed inside the shoe as a kind of insole. They can be prescribed under the National Health Service and are often very helpful. It is most important that the pad or 'metatarsal button' is placed in exactly the right place. All too often the pad is put where the supplier thinks it ought to be rather than where the patient needs it. Special systems exist for making shaped cork or composition insoles to meet each individual patient's requirements.

The problem about an insole or any other padding put in the shoe, is that it is bulky and the shoe is often already too tight because of foot swelling. It is nearly always necessary with a shaped insole in arthritis to make sure that the patient has larger shoes. Certain chiropodists and footwear manufacturers carry a stock of shoes that are especially deeply lasted so as to make room not only for the foot but also for the insole. This is an ideal solution for people with mild foot deformity.

4 Valgus supports. These can be bought ready-made or in a form that can be easily moulded into the shape that the individual requires, or they can be made individually out of moulded plastic. Their job is to enable the area between the heel and the big toe – known in lay terms as the instep – to take some weight. They are needed only in 'secondary flat-foot' which is due to disease of the joints in the foot. Unfortunately, they are also often supplied to young people with primary, but normal, flatfoot, in which case they lead to muscle wasting and weakness. The best kinds of valgus supports are individually moulded and are kept in exactly the right position. In general, rigid supports and pads are not as well tolerated by patients as supple or cushioned ones, and there is now a wide range made out of modern foam plastics or micro-cellular rubbers.

The role of the surgeon

All surgeons would agree that the prevention of deformities in the joints of the feet is much better than operations to correct them. Much can be done for severe deformities but no foot which has had an operation is as good as a normal foot. The complicated balance of the foot and the mechanism of the anterior and longitudinal arches cannot usually be restored by surgery and an operation to correct deformity may make another more likely.

For example, an operation for a painful bunion joint often results in a shortening as well as a straightening of the big toe. At the same time the surgeon frequently has to remove the small sesamoid bone – little pieces of bone which are placed inside the strong tendon to allow it to slide over the joint. These sesamoid bones form part of the normal anterior arch and it is on them that weight is taken in the normal foot. Removing them means damaging the arch so that although the immediate results of the operation may be good in that the patient has a straight toe and is able to wear normal shoes again, later the results all too frequently include the development of metatarsalgia because of damage to the anterior transverse arch.

Similarly, the removal of a single toe because it is cocked up and rubbing on the shoe is sometimes followed by the other toes getting displaced into the gap and in turn causing trouble.

Therefore, if an operation is planned for the forefoot, it either has to be very minor or very radical – one which will not upset, or one for which it is worth upsetting the whole balance of the anterior arch.

In the past the most successful operation for serious arthritis of the toe-base joints was to remove all the toes. This was a mutilating operation but it worked well and, of course, the feet could be hidden in normal shoes and a pad was placed in the toe area.

Nowadays, more advanced operations have been devised which result in the toes being brought back into line, the patient wearing a normal shoe and something of the original arch restored. There are variations on this operation, which is called 'forefoot arthroplasty' and in one of the most successful of these variations the operation is done from the sole of the foot. This means that not only are the patient's toes straight and the pain removed, but even the scar left by the incision, through which the surgeon corrected the deformity, is hidden.

Operations are also performed for trouble in the joints at the back of the foot, particularly if they are painful or collapsing. In such cases it is usually necessary to stiffen the joints, for it has been found that a rigid but painless joint is more helpful to the patient than a painful moving one. The surgeon will usually put the foot in a plaster-of-Paris boot for a while to see if immobilization relieves pain. If it does, and if pain recurs when the plaster-of-Paris boot is removed, he may well recommend internal fixation of the joint by an operation. Extra care is necessary, since the patient with a stiff ankle is unable to point her toes. She cannot then get the foot into a normal lace-up shoe and shoes with extra long openings have to be provided.

Shoes and appliances

Shoes made for deformed or crippled feet are known paradoxically as surgical shoes. 'Medical shoes' would be a better term, since there is usually no question of operation.

Traditionally, surgical shoes are made using craftsmen techniques. The craftsman or the fitter sees the foot for which the shoe is to be made; he measures it around the 'waist' of the foot and at various other points and he selects a wooden last which is the nearest to the patient's size. He then tacks pieces of leather on to the last and by sanding these down and shaping them, he can turn the standard last into a shape similar to the patient's foot. The insole and the upper shoe are stitched together over the last. The shoe is then ready for the first fitting. If it is too tight or too loose a fit, adjustments are made after which the sole and the heel are stitched and nailed on.

This is a lengthy, time-consuming process. One skilled craftsman working hard can only make about six pairs of shoes a week at most. If the craftsman is also to spend some time seeing the foot for which the shoe is being made – as he should do – his output is even lower. It is therefore not surprising that such shoes are extremely expensive. In order to keep the cost down, the wages paid to these craftsmen are low. This means, in turn, that there are now very few apprentices entering the trade.

In Britain, the National Health Service provides surgical shoes for patients who need them, free of charge, on the prescription of the appropriate consultant. But this service, valuable as it is, is in danger of collapsing because of the difficulties of supply. The main problem now is that too many of these shoes are made by craftsmen who never see the foot for which they are making the shoe. The patient may have to wait for up to six months for a pair of shoes and, in the case of patients with arthritis, there is a strong possibility that the foot will change before the shoe is finally provided so that it will not fit.

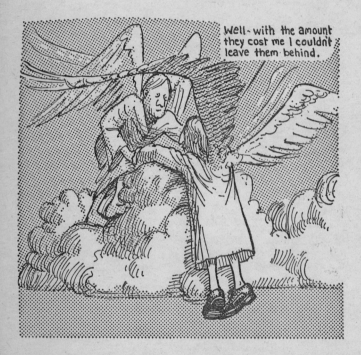

The traditional stitched and welted craftsman-shoe has another disadvantage. It is often very heavy. It dates from the days when lack of public and private transport necessitated walking, and shoes needed to be waterproof. But nowadays few people face the rain or the snow; they spend most of their lives indoors, in cars, trains or buses. This is particularly true of people with arthritis. Therefore a much lighter weight shoe is adequate, and preferable. The patient with arthritis of the knees cannot afford to have an extra pound weight on the feet by wearing heavy leather shoes when very lightweight plastic materials would be more appropriate.

What can be done? In many cases patients with mild deformities of the feet can buy shoes that fit from commercial sources. One firm in Britain makes especially wide shoes for people with hallux valgus that is not too severe. They also make women's shoes which have ornamental lacing right down to the toes; this allows for a considerable degree of modification in the shape of the shoe. Most shops now carry a stock of very cheap, light, soft plastic shoes which can look quite smart and do not press on bony prominences. Chiropodists can supply shoes that are deeply lasted so as to take a shaped or cushioned insole to look after deformities on the sole of the foot.

Also it seems that science has not ignored the importance of special shoes. Many hospitals are now using a modern and effective technique – known as the seamless shoe.

Seamless Shoes. Seamless shoes is the general name for shoes which are made by bonding rather than stitching techniques and are made directly to a modified plaster-of-Paris model of the patient's foot. They are derived from the so-called 'space shoes' which were invented in about 1940 in America, long before the Space Age. The original space shoe made no concessions to fashion. It was a foot-shaped shoe, very broad at the toes and very comfortable, but rather hot and sweaty in warm weather because it was made of impermeable materials.

The modern seamless shoe starts in the same way. The patient has a plaster-of-Paris case of the feet made. This cast is then sent to a manufacturer who fills up the cast with more plaster to reproduce the shape of the original foot. He then adds on extra plaster around the toes so as to make a last which is long enough for the toes to move forward during walking. He also narrows the last around the heel to ensure a snug heel fit. The difference between the modern seamless shoe and the 'space shoe' is that the insole only is made of lightweight micro-cellular rubbers or plastics, already moulded to the deformities of the patient's sole. The upper part of the shoe is not moulded but is made of very soft materials which will not rub. Lacing is still the best way of closing the shoe but for people who are unable to point the toes or whose fingers are arthritic and cannot manage laces, alternative methods such as a zip and ring are available. Such shoes can be very light, weighing only five or six ounces as opposed to twelve ounces for conventional surgical shoes. They can also be very durable – or at least they would be if they weren't put to so much use. The most durable shoes are those which are so uncomfortable that they are never worn!

Farmers and other outdoor workers who have foot problems can often wear their surgical shoes inside a large rubber overboot or snowboot. This gives almost as much protection as the conventional rubber boot and is certainly a lot warmer and more comfortable. Garage workers and other people who have their shoes exposed to oil have a special problem since oil and petrol have a bad effect on the special bonding agents used. Under such circumstances the shoe may fall to pieces. For them it is necessary to be sure that special oil-proof glues and cements are used in the manufacturing of the shoes. Workers in machine shops where there is a great deal of metal swarf have another sort of problem since modern shoe materials very easily pick up sharp metal fragments which work through the sole. Again, special care has to be taken. Such shoes need to be inspected daily and any pieces of metal splinters removed.

Given such precautions, the seamless shoe technique has been very successful. In one investigation, between eighty and ninety per cent of patients fitted by this method were satisfied and were able to wear their shoes at first fitting. This compares to the usual level of around fifty per cent for the traditional surgical shoe technique. And as conventional surgical shoes cost about twice as much, seamless shoes are cheaper as well as more convenient and effective.

11 Does rheumatism affect family life and sex life?

Some forms of rheumatism are chronic diseases persisting over many years and the doctor may have no alternative but to tell his patient to 'learn to live with it'. And learning to live with a rheumatic condition is just what many sufferers do with extra-

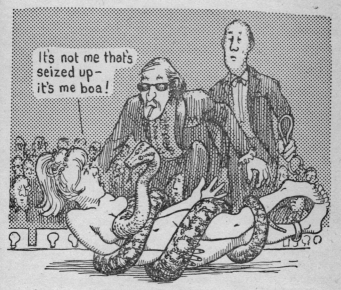

Learning to live with rheumatism

ordinary success, undefeated by what can often be a continuous nagging disability or for some, a long drawn out pain. In fact, it is these undaunted people who are best equipped to teach and reassure the other less confident sufferers.

It *is* possible to live with arthritis and rheumatism, to grow up, marry, to make love and to produce normal healthy children. But it can be hard sometimes, and inevitably people worry about some of the real, and apparent, problems that they will have to cope with. It is for those people that need reassurance that this chapter is intended. The main areas of concern are how rheumatism affects:

1 the lives of children and teenagers
2 having a family and the methods of contraception
3 pregnancy
4 making love.

How rheumatism affects the young

The child

Serious forms of rheumatism in children are very rare. Strangely, very young children tend to accept it psychologically more adequately than those who are affected in their teens. A toddler or a young child with bad joints who has to go to hospital and has to be kept in bed for a long time is often the centre of a great deal of care and attention. Within the family he may get more of his mother's concern than his fit brothers and sisters. At school or in hospital, not only are there many people to look after him, but often there are other children similarly affected. He is rarely deprived of 'extra' love and the discomfort he is experiencing in his own body is, to him, normal – he has never known any other condition. The much used saying 'What you've never had, you'll never miss' is not without relevance to the child who has suffered from a rheumatic condition since infancy. If the disease persists (and only a minority of forms do), it is possible for him to grow up having spent a long time away from school, perhaps even having had many operations and treatments and having failed to grow to a normal height, but still to feel completely normal within himself. Such children do not appear to have any more difficulty than others in adjusting to the inevitable turmoils of growing up.

The teenager

The problems of contracting a severe form of rheumatism are more serious for older children and teenagers.

For the boy, being unable to compete in games and outdoor activities can be seen as a catastrophe for his school and social life. It may cause him to become withdrawn and shy. For the girl, the belief that she might not be pretty may undermine her confidence and some girls with rheumatism go through bouts of depression that are often out of all proportion to the apparent problem, just as other children go through agonies of feeling inferior because they have a spotty face or some inherited blemish.

This type of reaction is so natural that sociologists have developed numerous theories to explain it. 'The Looking-Glass Self' is a widely accepted concept which argues that people react in accordance with their ideas about the 'image' they display to others. Thus, if a child *thinks* he is not intelligent, his work *will* be of a low standard. Similarly, a rheumatic child may become withdrawn because he believes he is not able to participate.

Parents and friends will do their best to help a disabled youth, but this can be self-defeating as it can create an attitude of reliance on others (and personal inadequacy) that could persist through life. It is better to encourage independence whilst simultaneously *reassuring* the child that help is available if necessary.

Sexual development

The awakening of sexuality in adolescence is a complicated and sometimes painful process in any child, and children with rheumatism are not exempt from this process. However, the age when menstruation begins for girls and pubic hair grows on boys and girls along with the other characteristic sexual developments for both is seldom affected. And apart from a very few exceptions, nor is their ultimate ability to become parents impaired.

Educational development

There is a danger for all children and teenagers with rheumatic conditions of missing school or training. Yet for them, education is doubly important – they may, after all, have to work with their heads rather than with their hands. So hospitals with special schools, schools for the handicapped, home tutors and parents who will help with teaching and training are invaluable. Later on, it may be possible for them to be educated at universities or technical colleges which have been designed to allow access for disabled students.

Having a family and planning it

Is it inherited?

One or two rare rheumatic diseases are definitely inherited. The best known of these is HAEMOPHILIA, the bleeding disease which also affects joints. Only men are affected but daughters or sisters can pass on the disease to their children.

Another very rare disease – OCHRONOSIS – is inherited. Children born into a family with ochronosis are unable to use one of the amino acids which is present in protein food. Instead, this substance gets turned into a black waste product which is lost partially in the urine, and partly is deposited in joints, damaging them.

If there is haemophilia or ochronosis in the family, there are special advisory centres which can provide information about the dangers of passing the condition on.

Most other rheumatic diseases are not inherited in this straightforward sense, but particular conditions do occur more frequently within families than the 'average' would lead us to expect. For example, in Chapter 7, GOUT was described as having a tendency to run in families, and yet there are more gouty sufferers who do *not* have a relative affected than who do. Similarly, there is a tendency for osteoarthrosis, particularly the type that affects the end joints of the fingers, to affect several members of one family. Again, rheumatic fever (a form of rheumatism that follows a throat infection) seems to be concentrated within certain families, but this may be because all the members of the family would risk catching the same infection. The possibility of inheriting rheumatoid arthritis is very small. It is such a common condition that it is to be expected that occasionally there is more than one patient in the same family. But in fact, it does occur a little more frequently in families than chance alone would suggest. The most one can say, is that while the disease itself is clearly not inherited, a tendency or predisposition to it might be. Certainly, a parent with rheumatoid arthritis who wants a child should in no way be deterred from having one. The chance of his or her child getting rheumatoid arthritis is very small; the chance of the child being absolutely normal is very great.

Family planning and contraception

The fertility of most rheumatism sufferers is completely normal. The only evidence of reduced fertility is for a rare disease called disseminated lupus erythematosus and very occasionally for some women who have or who are ultimately destined to get rheumatoid arthritis.

This means that family-planning measures are just as important for rheumatism sufferers as for others. Mechanical methods, such as the rubber sheath for men or the Dutch cap and spermicide for women may be difficult for those who have crippled fingers to manage. Clearly, in such circumstances, the fit partner can take the initiative. Many women with rheumatoid arthritis use the IUD or coil method (which has to be inserted by a doctor) or a hormonal contraceptive such as the Pill. From the medical point of view, both methods are acceptable and safe, and will not make the arthritis worse, or interfere with the other drugs used for alleviation of rheumatic pain. However, for patients receiving treatment with cortisone or other steroids it is advisable to avoid use of intra-uterine devices such as the coil. The Pill does sometimes, however, cause aching of the limbs in young women but it is not serious. The aching stops when the Pill is stopped and it has nothing to do with the rheumatoid arthritis.

Those who do not agree with artificial methods of contraception, and who do not want children, are best advised to abstain from intercourse or use the 'rhythm' method. In the latter, intercourse only takes place in the so-called, but often mis-called 'safe period'. However, this is not reliable. Periods often do not occur at absolutely regular intervals so that errors of timing occur; many unwanted pregnancies are a result of intercourse in the 'safe period'. Identification of the 'safe period' can be improved by the use of a temperature chart obtained by the woman measuring her temperature daily in the usual fashion. The alternative, *coitus interruptus* or premature withdrawal, is neither contraceptively safe nor psychologically sound and has little to commend it – it doesn't make good sex!

For the older person and once the family is complete, surgical sterilization is often the answer. It is a relatively minor procedure and is available for both men and women. However, do remember that it may be difficult and sometimes impossible to reverse the procedure should circumstances change and further children be desired.

Pregnancy and rheumatism

Pregnancy and rheumatoid arthritis

Pregnancy often brings about a temporary alleviation of rheumatoid arthritis. Welcome as this is, it can be something of a fool's paradise – within a few weeks and sometimes even within a few hours after the baby's birth, the condition returns to where it would have been if the woman had never been pregnant. This sometimes leads to the pregnancy being blamed as the cause of the rheumatoid arthritis, when the disease had previously been very mild or unnoticed.

Interestingly, it was the improvement during pregnancy which first convinced doctors that rheumatoid arthritis was a reversible condition and that research would one day find a permanent and harmless way of reversing it. A similar remission sometimes takes place in patients who develop jaundice. Dr Philip Hench postulated that in pregnancy there must be a 'Substance X' circulating in the blood which suppresses arthritis. We now know that this is so, and that the 'Substance X' is cortisol, a normal hormone and a form of cortisone produced in the adrenal glands. In pregnancy the mother is getting an extra dose of cortisol and in jaundice the liver, which gets rid of excess cortisol, fails to do so, so the amount in the blood increases. Unfortunately, the discovery did not lead to the hoped-for establishment of a total cure for rheumatoid arthritis. Cortisol and its many derivatives, of which the best known are cortisone, prednisone and prednisolone, are only a way of temporarily suppressing this disease, and (see Chapter 4) if used for a long time, they produce unpleasant side effects.

Pregnancy and back pain

Back pain does not necessarily mean that the pain is arising from the back. Sometimes a previous disease or displacement of one of the organs inside the abdomen or pelvis (including the womb in a woman) may be the cause of the complaint. So, because the position of other organs is altered when the baby is growing in the womb, pregnancy may either alleviate or increase this type of pain.

However, pain arising from the lower spine is often made worse by pregnancy, particularly when there has been a previous episode of prolapsed disc or when there is a minor inherited abnormality of the spine. Special spinal supports or postural exercises may be needed to ensure that the whole weight of the developing womb and the baby do not have to be entirely supported by a weak back. It is easy to forget that although the baby at birth may weigh eight or nine pounds, this is only half the weight of the total pregnant womb. Add to this the tendency for a pregnant woman to put on fat and to accumulate fluid with swelling of the ankles, and it is easy to see why mothers with weak backs feel pain due to carrying around such enormous extra burdens.

Pregnancy and rheumatic fever and heart disease

Happily, rheumatic fever and rheumatic heart disease are very rare conditions. But at one time, this was an important cause of death of the mother during pregnancy. In the later stages of pregnancy, and particularly during the birth process itself, the heart has to do a lot of extra pumping; rheumatic fever, when it affects the heart, damages the valves and makes the pumping action inefficient. The danger is such that in the past, women with bad hearts have been advised not to become pregnant, or if they do, to have an abortion and, possibly, be sterilized.

Sometimes this advice has led to bitter arguments, often on religious grounds. On the one side, there are those who believe that contraception, abortion and sterilization are wrong and, on the other side, there are those who think that the health, and possibly the very survival, of the mother, must come first. She is not much good to her first-born children if she dies in the process of presenting them with a brother or sister. Fortunately, these difficult emotional decisions can nowadays nearly always be avoided. Birth can be brought on early when the baby is not so big. Operations can be performed to correct damaged valves, even during pregnancy. Drugs are available to sustain the damaged heart and to correct heart failure before it gets too bad.

Pregnancy and hip disease
Stiff painful hips can make it difficult to part the legs and are then a serious problem in pregnancy. A natural birth may be impossible and a Caesarian (surgical) birth will usually be needed. This is also true when the sacroiliac joints which connect the spine to the pelvic bones behind the hips, are damaged. Their normal function is to allow the birth canal to expand to allow the baby to be born; if they cannot do this the birth passage will be too small for a natural birth.

Pregnancy relating to other forms of rheumatism
Pregnancy does not make any particular difference to other types of rheumatic conditions, many of which occur long after the age of childbirth anyway.

But there are two conditions which are actually caused by pregnancy – the carpal tunnel syndrome and sacroiliac strain.

In the *Carpal Tunnel Syndrome* the important median nerve which conducts messages from the skin of the thumb and adjacent three fingers becomes subject to pressure as it passes through the tunnel in the front of the wrist. Pregnancy can initiate this because it leads to a general increase of fluid in the limbs, which in turn can squash the nerve in its rather narrow tunnel. This pressure produces a tingling and burning sensation in the fingers which is especially troublesome at night. Fortunately, this clears up a week or two after the baby is born.

Sacroiliac Strain sometimes follows pregnancy. The sacroiliac joints spread open under the effect of a special birth hormone which relaxes and enlarges the birth passage. Each sacroiliac joint can be likened to the two parts of a scallop shell; because they are not smooth, when the two parts of the joint come together again, all the irregularities must fit exactly into each other. Occasionally there is a slight misfit and the pelvis tightens up with the joint in a strained position. A strong pelvic binder will often relieve any pain.

Making love

Even our Victorian grandparents, who would have found it difficult to discuss the subject of sex with any naturalness and freedom, would agree that if a principal purpose of marriage is bearing children and raising a family, then a normal sex life is essential. Today we go further and tend to stress the importance of a healthy sex life whether the couple desire to have children or not.

Do rheumatic diseases interfere with a couple's sex life? On the whole the answer is 'No', unless psychological factors interfere, with physical consequences.

First, what is a normal sex life? Some recent studies of human sexual love have concluded that anything is normal as long as it is practised by consenting adults. There is a great range and richness in attitudes to sex amongst men and women. The frequency of intercourse, the time of day, the circumstances, all differ remarkably; for some couples twice a day is normal,

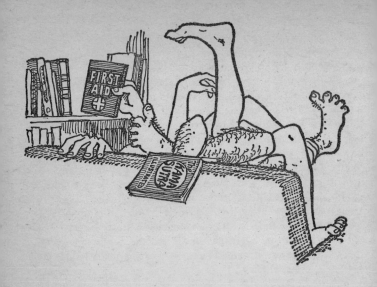

others once a month or less; some are only sexually aroused in the morning, others at night and in the dark. Just as there is a wide range of what is normal with regard to frequency, so there is a wide range as regards preliminaries. Some need an elaborate sex-play and ritual before making love, for others this is unnecessary.

Psychological factors

Arousal is a psychological process even though it has physical effects. The signs of sexual arousal are obvious in the male, and although not so obvious in the woman, they are just as important since this leads to the secretion of mucus which is the natural lubricant in the sexual act. How does rheumatism affect the patient psychologically?

Significantly, ninety per cent of the sex and marriage problems that affect couples where one or other has a rheumatic disease are exactly the same old problems that affect non-rheumatic people. They are the 'typical' problems that the

Marriage Guidance Clinics deal with every day. They are therefore 'normal problems' despite their immediate serious nature. Except in certain special circumstances, being a rheumatic sufferer does not mean that a person's marriage and sex life is bound to be a failure, or even particularly difficult.

For the man, arousal is often quick but nevertheless dependent on a psychological feeling that he is a man, and this means more than just being a man in bed. It is not always possible for the husband who has a serious form of arthritis to carry out his traditional role as the breadwinner, going out to work to provide for his family. Again sociologists have a term for this type of situation – 'role reversal'. The wife goes out to work whilst the husband, because of his disabilities, stays at home perhaps pottering about attempting to do some housework. Psychologically, the loss of role can be difficult for him and may be reflected in impotence unless both he and his wife understand the problem.

An often successful solution is for the man to develop a hobby or interest, perhaps learning the skills of something he previously wanted to do but never had time for. One traditional function of hospital occupational therapy departments is the teaching and encouragement of hobbies for those unable to work or who are past retirement age. The wife needs to understand the psychological importance of these outlets and to encourage them even though they may mean more work for her on top of her already full programme. Belittling the husband's hobby is to belittle him and may be reflected in impotence.

For the wife a psychological part of sexuality is display, or looking and feeling attractive, and if she feels attractive, she will be. Again, it is the concept of the looking-glass self; if she thinks her husband – and everybody else – finds her unattractive, she will act according to that belief. Attractive clothing, hair styles and make-up are important and if she cannot reach shops and hairdressers, special arrangements to bring these facilities to her home should be encouraged.

Surgery and arthritis of the hip
One of the welcome benefits of modern surgery for arthritis

of the hip is that it permits normal love-making again. With a couple, one of whom has hip disease, this may make all the difference between a happy and successful marriage and one in which the marriage is in danger of breaking up because sex is impossible.

Communicating from single beds?

It may seem to be a good idea when one person is in pain and having difficulty in sleeping, for the 'healthier' member of the couple to move from a double bed to a single bed, or even to a separate room. But – and this advice is not meant to sound patronizing – think carefully about it; much of marital love is based upon good communications, being able to talk to one another, touch each other and to lie together. For older people the sexual act itself is not essential, but sleeping apart may lead to isolation and to loss of contact both in the psychological as well as in the physical sense.

Some people find it convenient to make love after taking tablets for pain relief. Others feel so stiff in the early morning and so much better in the afternoon, that it is worth any extra effort needed to enable the couple to make love during the afternoon.

Further reading

Those who would like further advice on this subject are advised to write for the booklet 'Marriage, Sex and Arthritis' issued by the Arthritis & Rheumatism Council, 8–10 Charing Cross Road, London WC2H OHN.

12 Spas and spa therapy

Spa waters have always been associated with the treatment of rheumatism and arthritis. The belief in the inherent ability of natural waters to relieve rheumatic symptoms is one of the few remaining indications of the symbolism which has surrounded water through the past centuries – one has only to read the Bible to see that water was often thought to possess magical qualities for healing both soul and body. In classical mythology, certain waters also had the same types of powers. For example, there is the story of Prince Bladud and the pigs who were cured of leprosy by the hot waters of Bath. But the use of water as a healing agent is not confined to legend. The ancient physicians, Hippocrates, Celsus and Galen are known to have used it, and as a more obvious example, the Romans built large centres with pools designed partly for treatment and partly as places for relaxation. In Britain, the remains of a Roman spa have been uncovered in Bath and the pools and hot air chambers have been preserved and restored to an excellent state.

The fashionable development of spas
Spa treatment, like nearly everything else, has been the subject of whims of fashion. After the Romans left, spa treatment lapsed in Britain despite its popularity in the famous centres in Europe. Although sufferers have made pilgrimages to Buxton for many centuries it was not until the reign of Queen Elizabeth I that it became a fashionable resort for nobility and gentry to come to 'take the waters'. At that time, treatment consisted of simply taking a 'quick dip' in pools of hot mineral water and of drinking this water in large quantities. One technique reported was to begin with seven pints of water daily and increase this intake by one pint each day to a maximum of fourteen pints a day!

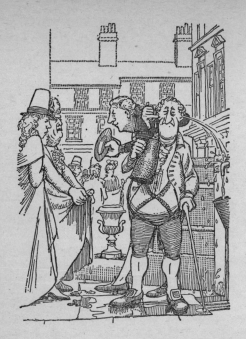

Bath only became fashionable as a spa centre when the city was rebuilt in the eighteenth century to the magnificent designs of John Wood and his son. This architectural masterpiece, with its open streets, splendid crescents and elegant buildings such as the Pump Room, led to the arrival of such nobility as Beau Nash and subsequently to development of the high status of Bath's society - as is depicted in Jane Austen's novels. As a result, Bath was probably the most fashionable centre for spa treatment in Britain during the eighteenth century, and had many famous physicians, such as Dr William Oliver - the inventor of the Bath Oliver Biscuit.

The medical development of spas

But at that time the attractions of Bath and of all the spa centres were as health resorts, cultural centres and places for relaxation as well as centres for medical treatment. In some cities the originally medical concept disappeared entirely, and today the recreational and amenity aspects are all that remain. In London, Sadler's Wells and Battersea Gardens are typical examples of watering places that have lost their medical flavour.

During the nineteenth century, however, other spas became less fashionable and recreational and more medically orientated. Many centres endeavoured to develop a scientific approach towards treatment and towards providing specific benefit for particular illnesses. Successful or beneficial treatment was claimed for many diseases which had little or no connection with rheumatism and arthritis, and the extravagance of some of these claims led to a more critical approach in assessing the value of spa therapy.

The modern spas were originally developed on the sites of natural springs providing water which contained a high mineral content. The chemical contents of these waters have been carefully analysed and found to remain remarkably constant at any particular centre. In some spas the waters are still hot as they emerge from the ground, and this is due to some subterranean volcanic activity. Some heat may be generated by the decay of radioactive materials in the earth's crust. Fortunately, very little of this radioactivity gets into the water that actually emerges.

The different kinds of spa waters – sulphurous, acid or alkaline, potable or containing salts to the constituency of strong brine, depend on the nature of the underground beds through which the water is forced before it reaches the surface.

Do spa waters relieve rheumatism?

We know that immersion in hot water not only allows the joints to move more readily but also produces alterations in the circulation of blood. Indeed the swollen joints may actually diminish in size. But the experiments to prove this were all done using tap water. Do the natural waters in spas have any further value ? Despite the past efforts to prove otherwise, the claims that have been made for particular waters being of value for specific illnesses have not been verified. For that matter however, scientists have not proven that these waters are of no value. A visit to almost any natural hot springs will show some remarkable features. At Rotorua in New Zealand, at Yellowstone in the United States and at Bath in England, the water comes out of the ground far too hot to touch – almost at boiling heat in some springs. Yet in this hot water, as soon as it is exposed to the light, certain organisms grow. They are known as thermophilic bacteria and they can withstand temperatures which boil an egg. They are thought to be the relics of the first primitive organisms on earth before it cooled down. If there is any life on Venus it could be this kind of organism. They grow on the surface of the water and on the muddy sides of the hot pools producing red, green and yellow scum. Could they be producing any marvellous substance which is good for relieving rheumatic diseases ? It doesn't seem likely but scientists cannot at this moment rule it out. But even if there is no inherent healing quality in these waters, spa centres can provide the best sort of environment for treating rheumatism. The warm waters can be used for hydrotherapy and, more important, the actual atmosphere of the spa centre is psychologically beneficial.

Psychological relaxation

Spas are usually in sunny sheltered towns protected from the extremes of the weather. They are often surrounded by beautiful countryside and have magnificent parks and gardens with planned walks that will introduce the patients to splendid views. In addition to this, most spa towns, as a result of their cultural heritage, can boast of theatres, concert halls, exhibition halls, restaurants, and elegant historic buildings, which stand to this day and are still used and enjoyed. The psychological value of such a setting is obvious: the patient can make a break from the stresses and strains of his normal life – and just relax! Freedom from worry about work and home combine with the intrinsic benefits of spa centres to produce this psychological relaxation. The popularity of the spas becomes easy to understand.

Spa treatments

Hydrotherapy. Hydrotherapy is the term applied to the use of water as a means of treatment. The physiotherapists who employ this technique are termed 'hydrotherapists'. Not surprisingly, therefore, physical treatment in the spa revolves around the hydrotherapy department.

The main value of using water – whether it is spa water or ordinary tap water – is that in it the body weighs considerably less. This physical principle was first enunciated by Archimedes when he showed that the weight of any object in water is decreased by an amount equal to the weight of water displaced by that body – which is the same principle that allows us to swim. This means in reference to treating rheumatism, that a patient immersed in a pool need only exert a small amount of effort to support his body. Damaged joints can easily be put through a wide range of movements so that weak muscles can be strengthened. Hot water will relieve spasm in muscles and help them to function more efficiently.

Treatment is usually carried out in a large pool of varying depth so that the patient is immersed to the appropriate extent. Especially for hip problems is the Hubbard tank in which exercises are performed under water and the hydrotherapist can treat the patient without having to enter the pool herself.

Exercises. It is in the restoration of movement and muscle power that the spas probably provide their greatest benefits for arthritic patients. In severe arthritis, it is the hydrotherapist who puts in the effort to move the joints whilst the patient lies relaxed in the warm bath. But, for the lesser and more common degrees of rheumatism and aches and pains, there is far greater value in the patient using his own muscle power.

Local stimulation to the skin is performed by a wide variety of techniques, to relieve pain in particular areas. A douche or spray of water under pressure may be applied directly to the painful area and is sometimes combined with massage. Also used in some places are aerated baths, foam baths and brine baths.

Massage is an adjunct to hydrotherapy and exercises, particularly for relieving spasm. It may be performed either in or out of the water or even whilst under a spray. But as the earlier reference to massage in this book suggested, its true value is rather doubtful.

Mud baths. Mention of spa treatment often elicits the response 'Oh, that's where you get mud baths'. There is a belief that different forms of mud, peat or hot sand possess special qualities for relieving rheumatic pains. The reputations of the great European spa centres were largely derived on this basis. These ideas have been fostered by the practitioners of mud treatment but there is no evidence to suggest that it is of any greater benefit

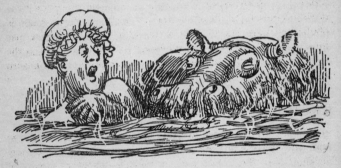

than merely being a useful method of applying local heat. These baths – no longer used in Britain – are prepared by mixing the mud or peat with water and heating the mixture to the required temperature with a jet of steam. The patient lies in the bath for perhaps fifteen minutes or half an hour and is later removed, showered off, wrapped in hot towels and allowed to sweat freely. In Britain we do sometimes use the mud pack, in which hot mud is enclosed in a bag and placed directly on the painful joint or on the back. Aesthetically, this seems much more acceptable. The combination of stimulation of the senses by heat, touch, and pressure is particularly relaxing for muscles tensed up by pain.

Electrotherapy refers to the types of treatment in which heat is applied to the limbs with electrical apparatus. They are 'no touch' techniques in that the apparatus does not come into direct contact with the patient. By short-wave diathermy the heat is generated in the tissues under the skin, whereas by infrared radiation it is applied to the skin surface only.

All methods of local heating relieve pain – possibly because messages of heat and pain compete for the same nerves in the nervous system and these cannot transmit both types of message at once. The relief lasts for about half an hour after the treatment and this give the physiotherapist a chance to get otherwise stiff or painful limbs moving again without hurting the patient.

There is another way of using electricity and that is by a series of tiny (and not very unpleasant) electrical shocks over the nerves to muscles to make the muscles contract. This method is often used most successfully in teaching patients how to use muscles they have forgotten they ever had. The muscles in the feet are an example; they may need to be retrained in people with foot strain.

The decline of the old spas

In the last few years the attitude of the medical profession to spas and spa therapy has radically altered. Medicine is now seeking more direct evidence of the benefits of all forms of treatment and of the positive value of any particular therapy employed. By and large this has been lacking in many continental spa centres, where many of the trappings used are merely 'holiday luxuries'. But there are honourable exceptions, and some of the great spa centres in Europe (as in Britain) have made outstanding contributions to the scientific study and the medical treatment of rheumatic diseases. Before journeying to a spa, the sufferer should seek expert advice on which spa is medically acceptable and not just a medically flavoured holiday resort. In Britain, spas have been closed down. In Europe, spas are booming. In Britain, they were largely run by the National Health Service. In France, and some other countries, they are run by the Government Tourist Agencies. Could there be a connection?

For this reason, the influence of the traditional spas in Britain has waned. Bath was one of the few remaining spas to remain in use, but even there the City Council has now closed the old treatment centre.

Modern treatment centres are being developed in which the emphasis is on the specific medical treatment of the disease combining drug treatment, surgery and physical treatment in one programme.

The disappearance of the spa is for many a sad farewell to an age of elegance in medicine, which is no longer fashionable.

Although there have been great advances in the treatment of rheumatic diseases, these may have been at the expense of treating the patient as a whole personality rather than as a collection of medical problems.

13 Acupuncture, herbalism and folk medicine

Arthritis and rheumatism have been described as diseases that produce 'long pain'. Most of the conditions described in this book are recurrent, persistent and irritating; patients really do have to be 'long suffering' in the face of conditions which do not kill but for which there is no real or absolute cure.

The search for help

Through orthodox means ...

Treatment and relief is normally sought by visits to the family doctor or hospital, but unfortunately snags can occur because of the very nature of these chronic diseases. The initial confidence in the doctor – who can usually take steps to relieve the pain – may wear off over a long period of time if there is little evidence of a dramatic change or improvement. Patients may feel that the doctor is losing interest in them and, even more disturbing perhaps, there may be a feeling of loss of continuity in medical care; doctors, particularly in hospitals, change their jobs frequently, and so a patient visiting at six-monthly intervals may hardly ever see the same doctor twice. Consequently, each new doctor may fail to get to grips with his or her particular problem. These criticisms of our profession will – hopefully – soon be no longer valid. In the past few years there has been a significant increase of interest by the medical profession in arthritis and rheumatism with a consequent improvement in the standard of medical care. Administrative attempts are being made to ensure that patients do see the same doctor on each consultation.

... and via less orthodox ways

It is partly this situation which has encouraged some people with rheumatism or arthritis to seek advice and help outside the medical profession. Any apparent lack of interest by the doctor in these 'persistent' conditions is often fully compensated for by well meaning friends and acquaintances, who may recommend consulting unorthodox 'healers' or trying various 'natural' remedies.

Folk remedies have been used for many different diseases. In particular, folklore thrives and flourishes in the type of chronic disease that persists for many years and varies in severity – such as arthritis. The natural course of these afflictions is not one of continuous and everlasting pain, but a changeable pattern in which the symptoms disappear and reappear for no particular reason. If folk remedies are taken and coincide with a 'disappearance' of the symptoms, then whatever is being taken at the time naturally tends to get the credit. The big snag is that it won't work for someone else or even for the same person next time.

Assessing the value of drugs

The problem of assessment of a particular drug or type of medical treatment is more difficult than one would assume. It is easy to be misled – many of the traditional medical remedies made no difference to the disease that they were supposedly curing or helping. Several factors can influence or bias an opinion as to whether a drug is useful or not.

1 The new medicine is not an isolated factor. Symptoms may come and go unrelated to the particular treatment being tested. To give an over-simple example: there is no known remedy which will kill the germs responsible for the common cold, but if a doctor said 'Remedy x will cure your cold in ten days' time', he could claim that 'Remedy x' was successful, for obviously you are unlikely still to have the same cold ten days later.

2 If drugs are presented in the right way and the patient believes that they will do some good, this treatment is likely to make him feel better. This is the so-called 'placebo reaction': the new remedy produces an improvement purely because of the belief that it will do so – it is a psychological improvement. This reaction is precisely why witch doctors have been – and still are –

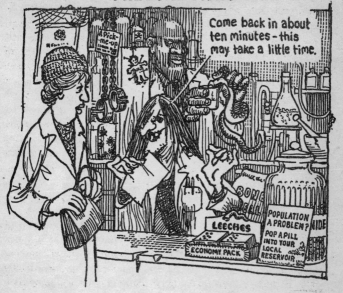

successful in some parts of the world. Both situations encourage a 'self-fulfilling prophecy'.

The psychological force must never be underestimated as it can and does elicit improvements. For example, patients with angina or heart pain may be unable to walk more than say, a hundred yards. But when a placebo agent is first tried, they may be able to walk double that distance before they feel severe pain. Unfortunately this psychological benefit never lasts for very long.

3 The physical appearance of the drug is another factor which creates bias. Research has shown that the way in which the tablets, capsules or mixtures actually appear, affects the patient's response. Unpleasant tasting medicines are thought by some patients to be more effective than those which are either tasteless or can be enjoyed, even though the actual drug contained within

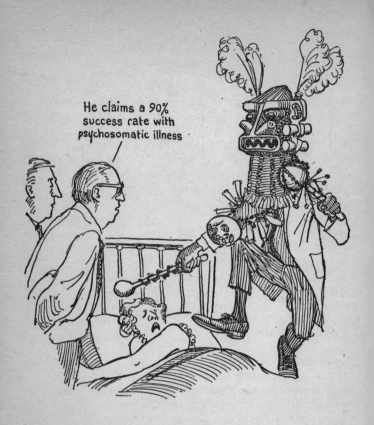

them is identical! Even the use of different coloured tablets and capsules can provoke a biased response.

The Victorian physicians seemed to be aware of this, for their policy – which was probably subconscious rather than deliberate – laid emphasis on the use of elegant preparations of medicines which in themselves were not very effective.

4 The patient's desire to please the doctor may influence his opinion of a new drug. When a patient feels that the doctor has taken a special interest in him and, instead of just leaving a prescription with the receptionist, goes out of his way to consult the patient and look for the most suitable drug, it is not surprising that he is more likely to feel that this drug is doing good.

5 Doctors can be equally misled when assessing the responses of patients. If the physician is enthusiastic, doing his utmost to help and is convinced that the drugs are useful, then he is more likely to 'see' and record benefit for a patient who has been following his advice.

Today, the medical profession is fully aware of these difficulties of assessment and of the need for careful testing to make sure that new drugs really do work. The only way in which the true benefits of a drug are ascertained is by the 'double-blind controlled trial'. This test is applied by giving the new medicine to one group of patients and a drug of proven value is given to another group. Neither the patients nor the doctors know who is receiving the standard drug or the new drug and so the progress of the patients is assessed without bias. Both patients and doctors are studying the effects of the drug 'blind'. The key to who has been receiving which drug is held by a third party and at the end of the study the code is broken and careful statistical assessments are made to prove or dispute the value of the new remedy. It is only via this method that advances in the treatment of rheumatism and arthritis can occur.

Folk medicine and herbalism

The 'double-blind controlled trial' has never been used by the proponents of folk medicine, herbal remedies or acupuncture, so that the real value of their methods has never been scientifically tested.

That is not to say, however, that all of their remedies are useless. Many of the standard drugs used in medicine today were originally obtained from plants and have been used as herbal remedies through the centuries. For example, the foxglove, or to use its botanical name, 'digitalis lanata' is an extremely poisonous flower which was given for centuries by folk medicine practitioners as a heart stimulant. William Withering then brought it into standard medical use in the eighteenth century and an extract from this plant, digitalis, is still perhaps the most useful single drug for patients with heart failure. Similarly, an extract from the Autumn Crocus was, for centuries, the only specific pain-relieving remedy for gout. It is still used – in a rather more sophisticated form as colchicine – for gout sufferers.

But although there is always the chance that new drugs may be discovered from the actual ingredients of a particular form of folk medicine, so far most have turned out to be valueless old wives' tales.

Numerous plant extracts are used for folk remedies, but there rarely appears to be any rhyme or reason as to why one is chosen rather than another. The use of such extracts thrives in the attitude of what is *natural* is also *good for you*, a belief which was as strong in past centuries as it is in the 'anti-pollution' ethos of today. Quite what 'natural' and 'good for you' really mean is hard to say. The wide variety of extracts used implies that they are of little help – if one or two were really useful, they would be used to the exclusion of all the others.

Apple Cider Vinegar is a popular folk lore remedy for arthritis. It is based on the belief that somehow the acid helps to digest food and makes the tissues of the body more tender, thereby reducing stiffness. Interesting as it may be to speculate on this theory, there is in fact no evidence to support it, particularly as there is only a small amount of acid present in apple cider vinegar, and only a fraction of what is naturally formed by the body itself within the stomach! There is no possibility that this small amount of acid could make any difference to digestion or to the body tissues.

Those who swear by apple cider vinegar probably gain psychological rather than physical relief. A story to support this is that of a devotee of apple cider vinegar who visited North Carolina – where it is the standard type of vinegar sold in the shops – and discovered that when it was freely available, it no longer seemed to be doing him any good!

Honey could perhaps be described as a herbal remedy of better taste! All the different types of honeys have their unique flavours (as well as being a good source of calories), but again

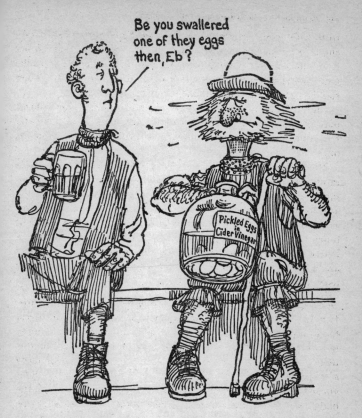

there is no evidence that honey alters the course of rheumatism and arthritis.

Ointments and Liniments are traditional remedies for aches and pains. 'Rubbing something in' provides relief, but whether it is the 'rubbing' or the 'something' is unclear. Firmly rubbing a liniment in massages the underlying tissues and often relieves the muscle spasm which produces aches and pains. Liniments and ointments open up the blood vessels of the skin – producing redness or erythema – and this local improvement to the blood supply may be helpful in relieving pains.

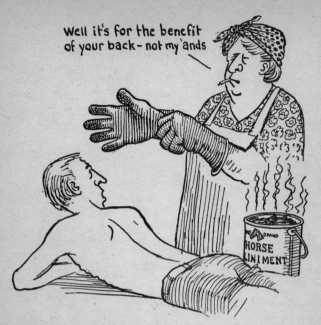

Standard liniment remedies can be purchased from the chemist's shop but there are many herbal remedies which exponents claim to be more effective. Traditional materials recommended are camphor, dry mustard and oils, but more bizarre concoctions that are supposedly used are made by dissolving live earthworms and ants. The results are no doubt quite magical!

Baths are used in spa therapy and certainly hydrotherapists know how to draw the maximum benefit from them. Folk medicine has also developed its own assortment of baths which usually consists of adding herbs to the bath water. Again, however, there are some bizarre ideas. One practitioner has recommended the use of ant baths and even suggested applying live ants around the painful joint so as to bite the skin. Such treatment (in many ways reminiscent of sixteenth century medicine) sounds rather more like a test of faith than profitable advice.

A Copper Bracelet for relieving rheumatism is probably the most popularly accepted myth. The misinformed argument behind this old wives' tale is that copper removes the electricity from the body. If a patient believes in his bracelet, then there is no reason for him to stop wearing it, but it is sad to see a clinic full of people badly affected by rheumatoid arthritis steadfastly wearing their copper bracelets – a fact which is evidence in itself of their 'irrelevance'. A reason for the widespread commercial support for this particular folklore may not be entirely unrelated to the fact that these bracelets are made from copper costing a few pence and are usually sold for £1 or more.

Associated with the belief in copper bracelets removing electricity from the body is the tenet that many present day rheumatic problems are due to the wearing of SHOES. Shoes, it is said, insulate the feet from the ground so that electricity is retained within the body. There are even stories of people who attach one end of a wire to the leg and trail the other behind on the ground so as to discharge this build-up of electricity.

Acupuncture

Acupuncture can perhaps be described as the Chinese equivalent of our folk medicine. In recent years it has hit the news head-lines in a number of fascinating reports which explain how this unusual system of medicine, steeped in Chinese history, is now spreading to the Western civilization. Treatment involves in-serting tiny gold and silver needles under the skin at certain definite points relating to the particular disease. This sounds unpleasant, but according to those who administer treatment based on acupuncture, the process causes no pain and produces a cure.

There is no scientific proof that acupuncture provides any positive benefits for arthritis other than the psychological ones which are to be expected. It may be that the acupuncturists induce some form of hypnotic state in their patients so that at the time they believe themselves to be cured.

There is another possible explanation of how acupuncture might work which has only recently received attention from medical scientists and the acupuncturists themselves. It is well known that soldiers in action on the battlefield may deny having any pain despite major injuries which normally would require injections of morphine. There must be some mechanism within the brain which prevents the sensation of pain reaching consciousness. This is the basis of the 'gate control theory' of how the feeling of pain is prevented. An inhibiting mechanism is operated – the gate is closed – so that pain is no longer experienced. The psychological stimulus of a battlefield, rubbing the skin over a bruise or stimulating certain nerves with the acupuncturist's needles, may suppress the sensation of pain in this way. Operations are said to be performed in China using acupuncture instead of conventional anaesthesia, and perhaps this is how it works – when it works. It certainly does not work in everybody, as even the Chinese admit.

But both hypnosis and the gate control mechanism of preventing pain are essentially short-term manoeuvres and can do nothing to cure rheumatism and arthritis.

In conclusion

At first sight the rather extraordinary and sometimes monstrous methods used in folk medicine appear amusing, but at a deeper level it is sad that patients should have to resort to these measures. It is only natural that a patient should seek help for him or herself. This is particularly so for sufferers with rheumatism and arthritis because their symptoms are chronic and recurrent and although a lot of help may be derived from the types of medical treatment described earlier in this book, patients may nevertheless be left with unpleasant symptoms. An understanding of the causes, processes and treatment involved in the various types of rheumatism is important to the sufferer – which is why this book was written – but a realistic account will give no unrealistic promises. Unorthodox remedies, often very expensive and presented in an elegant fashion, inspire a belief in their ability to do good. It is likely – and understandable – that these types of remedies will persist until the day comes when medical science finds a real cure for arthritis and rheumatism.

Appendix Organizations concerned with arthritis or rheumatism

It is not possible to give a comprehensive list of all the various charitable and other organizations concerned with the problems of arthritis and rheumatism. There are many local societies which provide invaluable help within the particular area in which they are situated and these have not been included.

The following list includes details of national societies concerned with the welfare of disabled or arthritic people, organizations for the dissemination of information about advances in treatment of arthritis and rheumatism and raising charitable funds to further research, and scientific societies for doctors and other research workers studying the rheumatic diseases.

Arthritis & Rheumatism Council (Empire Rheumatism Council)
8–10 Charing Cross Road, London WC2H OHN
A charitable organization which finances research into arthritis and rheumatic diseases. The Council also provides an information service to medical practitioners to keep them abreast of recent advances in the treatment of arthritis, and publishes booklets on various diseases for the use of patients.

British Association of Rheumatology and Rehabilitation
Royal College of Physicians, Regent's Park, London NW1 4LE
A scientific organization for physicians practising rheumatology and rehabilitation.

British Council for Rehabilitation of the Disabled
Tavistock House (South), Tavistock Square, London WC1
An educational and advisory body for disabled people.

British Orthopaedic Association
Royal College of Surgeons of England, 35–43 Lincoln's Inn Fields, London WC2A 3PN

An association for surgeons and physicians concerned with the advancement of the science and art of orthopaedic surgery.

The British Red Cross Society

9 Grosvenor Crescent, London SWIX 7EJ

Provides a wide variety of services for handicapped people. In particular, they supply many different aids to help the disabled and publish a very useful catalogue listing what is available.

British Rheumatism and Arthritis Association

I Devonshire Place, London WIN 2BD

A welfare organization to provide information, advice and practical aid for those afflicted by the rheumatic diseases.

Central Council for the Disabled

34 Eccleston Square, London SWI

A central coordinating council concerned with the general welfare of the disabled.

Disabled Drivers' Association

4, Laburnham Avenue, Wickford, Essex

Concerned with protecting the welfare of the disabled and assisting and encouraging them to greater mobility.

Disabled Drivers' Motor Club Ltd

39 Templewood, Ealing, London WI3 8BU

Provides services and advice for disabled drivers.

Disabled Living Foundation

346 Kensington High Street, London WI4 8NS

Maintain a permanent display of a comprehensive range of aids for disabled people and supply full information on where they can be obtained. They act as an information service and supply regular up-to-date bulletins and will answer any inquiries. They also publish many booklets providing advice for the disabled.

Disablement Resettlement Officers

At the Employment Exchanges these officers provide advice and help in settling disabled people in appropriate employment. They maintain a register of disabled people for whom there are certain designated jobs. They can also arrange training in industrial rehabilitation units, government training centres, residential training centres, commercial colleges, and factories as appropriate.

Heberden Society

8–10 Charing Cross Road, London WC2H OHN

A scientific organization for physicians, surgeons and research workers concerned with all aspects of rheumatic diseases.

Industrial Rehabilitation Units

There are 25 units throughout the country run by the Department of Employment. They will assess a disabled individual's potential and aptitude and organize courses aimed at resettling him in employment. Admission to an Industrial Rehabilitation Unit is normally on the advice of the Disablement Resettlement Officer.

'Invalids at Home'
23 Farm Avenue, London NW2
A charitable organization aimed to help permanent invalids to live at home in greater comfort and security.

National Ankylosing Spondylitis Society
The Royal National Hospital for Rheumatic Diseases, Upper Borough Walls, Bath
A self-help society for patients with ankylosing spondylitis, their family and friends.

The National Fund for Research into Crippling Diseases
Vincent House, 1a Springfield Road, Horsham, Sussex
A charitable organization collecting and distributing funds for research into all types of crippling diseases.

PHAB Clubs (Physically Handicapped and Able Bodied)
30 Devonshire Street, London WIN 2AP
Is concerned with the integration of physically handicapped and able bodied young people in the community by running several residential training courses throughout the year. They are affiliated to the National Association of Youth Clubs and the Central Council for the Disabled.

Remploy Ltd
415 Edgware Road, Cricklewood, London NW2 6LR
A government sponsored organization for the employment of severely disabled people. It maintains many factories throughout the country.

Residential training centres for the disabled
Queen Elizabeth Training College for the Disabled
Leatherhead, Surrey

St Loye's College for the Training and Rehabilitation of the Disabled
Exeter

The Portland Training College for the Disabled
Harlow Wood, Mansfield, Notts

Finchale Training College for the Disabled
Durham

These are run by voluntary organizations providing courses lasting about six months to return disabled people to employment. Admission to these courses is normally obtained through the Disablement Resettlement Officer.

Sheltered Workshops
Cheshire Homes
7 Market Mews, London WIY 8HP

Cripplecraft Home
Strode Park, Herne Bay, Kent

Dorincourt Residential Sheltered Workshop
Oaklawn Road, Leatherhead, Surrey

Enham Village Centre
Andover, Hants

Forces Help Society and Lord Roberts Workshops
118–122 Brompton Road, London SW3
(for ex-service-men and women)

Horder Centres for Arthritics
Crowborough, East Sussex

John Groome's Association for the Disabled
Edgware Way, Edgware, Middlesex AG8 8YT

Papworth Village Settlement
Papworth Everard, Cambridge CB3 8RF

Will provide rehabilitation, training and permanent sheltered employment and some residential accommodation for disabled people.

Winged Fellowship Trust (Holidays for the Disabled)
79–80 Petty France, London SW1
Maintains holiday homes for the disabled in Chigwell, Essex and
Redhill, Surrey.

The Wingfield Trust
24 Station Road, Epping
A voluntary organization to help physically handicapped children and
young people to overcome their disabilities through the playing of
musical instruments and other activities.

Index

D. C. Jarvis MD
Arthritis & Folk Medicine 70p

When folk medicine swept through Britain and America with its amazing message of relief from countless diseases, the author received innumerable letters from sufferers from arthritis, lumbago, gout and muscular rheumatism, inquiring what Folk Medicine had to offer them for their misery.

Now Dr Jarvis replies – explaining step by step a simple, sensible method of treatment, evolved through generations of trial and error by the rugged folk of his native Vermont and meticulously tested against his own medical experience.

Folk Medicine 90p

The tough, hard-living mountain folk of the state of Vermont have a time-honoured folk medicine.

The late Dr Jarvis, a fifth generation native of Vermont, lived and practised among these sturdy people for over fifty years. This book is the result of his deep study of their way of life and in particular of their concepts of diet. These he was able to test against his formal medical training and prove by long experience.

He offers a new theory on the treatment and prevention of a wide variety of ailments – the common cold, hay fever, arthritis, high blood pressure, chronic fatigue, overweight and many others – and holds out a promise of zestful good health for young and old.

Dr Felix Mann
Acupuncture: Cure of Many Diseases £1

Today thousands of European and Russian doctors practise acupuncture in conjunction with Western medicine. In this fascinating and illuminating book Dr Felix Mann dispels the mystique of this ancient science and art, explaining in clear and easy terms its origins, theory and practice.

'Let us hope that Dr Felix Mann will succeed in persuading his colleagues and the public that the method produces good results'
ALDOUS HUXLEY

Dr Andrew Stanway
Taking the Rough with the Smooth 70p

The discovery that foods rich in dietry fibre (roughage) can help prevent the serious diseases of the affluent society has been heralded as the medical breakthrough of the decade. This is the definitive book on the subject written for the general reader.

Mouthwatering high-fibre recipes are included to enable readers to adapt their diets for a happier and healthier life.

Dr A. Ward Gardner and Dr Peter J. Roylance
New Essential First Aid £1

An easy-to-read, copiously illustrated handbook of first aid.

Completely up to date, and written in the light of the tremendous advances in surgery, and in resuscitation, the book shows clearly and simply how to carry out the correct actions in the right order.

'The authors have approached the subject of essential first aid in a new, interesting and sensible way, placing emphasis throughout on life-saving, speed and commonsense' *Dr A. Lloyd Potter in his Foreword*

Dr Barbara Evans
Life Change 80p

For every woman undergoing the change of life, Dr Evans, Managing Editor of *World Medicine*, explains what is happening to your body, your emotions and your relationships: how the menopause affects you; how to cope with it; how and when hormone treatment can help; sex and the menopause; the risks of cancer. This book brings knowledge, expertise and hope to those suffering the physical and psychological problems of the menopause.

Samuel Dunkell MD
Sleep Positions £1

A startling new perspective on our world of sleep, offered by an
eminent psychiatrist. In this captivating and remarkable book he lists
and names the various positions taken up by the sleeping body, and
shows how you can identify your own bedtime habits and understand
how they reveal all kinds of intriguing personality secrets.

'A convincing thesis' SUNDAY EXPRESS

'What fun to be able to tap your partner in the middle of the night
and say: "Excuse me, your sleep is showing" ' EVENING NEWS

Col James L. Anderson and Martin Cohen
The West Point Fitness and Diet Book £1.20

From the US Army's top experts in physical fitness – a complete
conditioning programme for every member of the family, enabling
each member to enjoy the best of health and top physical condition
whether they're involved in competitive sport, relaxing in
retirement, or busy at the office or in the home all day. Includes: the
walk/run plan – weight control and nutrition – posture: how to look
good – sports for everyone at every age – special fitness for women.